New Developments in Medical Research

Human Anatomy and Physiology

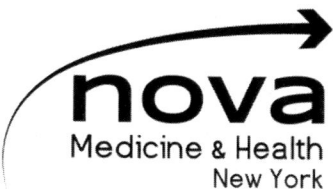

New Developments in Medical Research

A Literature Review on the Benefits of Propolis
Erik G. Martin (Editor)
2022. ISBN: 979-8-88697-253-5 (Softcover)
2022. ISBN: 979-8-88697-312-9 (eBook)

Autoimmunity and Cancer
Soner Şahin, PhD (Editor)
Kenan Demir, MD (Editor)
2022. ISBN: 978-1-68507-937-6 (Hardcover)
2022. ISBN: 979-8-88697-077-7 (eBook)

Bioprinting the Human
Soner Şahin, PhD (Editor)
Kenan Demir, MD (Editor)
2022. ISBN: 978-1-68507-993-2 (Hardcover)
2022. ISBN: 979-8-88697-066-1 (eBook)

Botulinum Toxin: Therapeutic Uses, Procedures and Efficacy
James C. Lark (Editor)
2022. ISBN: 978-1-68507-817-1 (Hardcover)
2022. ISBN: 978-1-68507-826-3 (eBook)

Astrocytes and Their Role in Health and Disease
Tomaz Velnar, MD, PhD (Editor)
Lidija Gradisnik, PhD (Editor)
2022. ISBN: 978-1-68507-983-3 (Softcover)
2022. ISBN: 979-8-88697-094-4 (eBook)

More information about this series can be found at
https://novapublishers.com/product-category/series/new-developments-in-medical-research/

Thomas Nordström

The Theoretical Foundation of Medicine

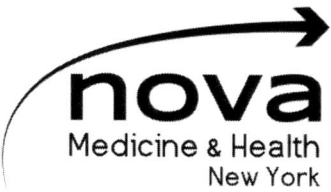

Copyright © 2023 by Nova Science Publishers, Inc.

https://doi.org/10.52305/TWHO5119

All rights reserved. No part of this book may be reproduced, stored in a retrieval system or transmitted in any form or by any means: electronic, electrostatic, magnetic, tape, mechanical photocopying, recording or otherwise without the written permission of the Publisher.

We have partnered with Copyright Clearance Center to make it easy for you to obtain permissions to reuse content from this publication. Simply navigate to this publication's page on Nova's website and locate the "Get Permission" button below the title description. This button is linked directly to the title's permission page on copyright.com. Alternatively, you can visit copyright.com and search by title, ISBN, or ISSN.

For further questions about using the service on copyright.com, please contact:
Copyright Clearance Center
Phone: +1-(978) 750-8400   Fax: +1-(978) 750-4470   E-mail: info@copyright.com

NOTICE TO THE READER

The Publisher has taken reasonable care in the preparation of this book, but makes no expressed or implied warranty of any kind and assumes no responsibility for any errors or omissions. No liability is assumed for incidental or consequential damages in connection with or arising out of information contained in this book. The Publisher shall not be liable for any special, consequential, or exemplary damages resulting, in whole or in part, from the readers' use of, or reliance upon, this material. Any parts of this book based on government reports are so indicated and copyright is claimed for those parts to the extent applicable to compilations of such works.

Independent verification should be sought for any data, advice or recommendations contained in this book. In addition, no responsibility is assumed by the Publisher for any injury and/or damage to persons or property arising from any methods, products, instructions, ideas or otherwise contained in this publication.

This publication is designed to provide accurate and authoritative information with regard to the subject matter covered herein. It is sold with the clear understanding that the Publisher is not engaged in rendering legal or any other professional services. If legal or any other expert assistance is required, the services of a competent person should be sought. FROM A DECLARATION OF PARTICIPANTS JOINTLY ADOPTED BY A COMMITTEE OF THE AMERICAN BAR ASSOCIATION AND A COMMITTEE OF PUBLISHERS.

Additional color graphics may be available in the e-book version of this book.

Library of Congress Cataloging-in-Publication Data

ISBN: 979-8-88697-460-7

Published by Nova Science Publishers, Inc. † New York

To all those fantastic people who work within medicine

Contents

Prologue		ix
Acknowledgments		xiii
Introduction		xv
Chapter 1	Postulates	1
Chapter 2	The Principle of Relations	5
Chapter 3	The Principle Applied to the Human Body	11
Chapter 4	DNA Transforms Masses	17
Chapter 5	The Lowest Common Denominator of Diseases	23
Chapter 6	The Scientific Illusion of Homeostasis	27
Chapter 7	How Mass Moves in the Human Body	39
Chapter 8	The Principle Applied to ATP Synthase and Sodium-Potassium Pump	63
Chapter 9	The Principle Applied to Inflammation and Its Diseases	75
Chapter 10	The Principle Applied to Cancer	83
Chapter 11	The Principle Applied to Testicular Cancer	97
Chapter 12	The Principle Applied to Alzheimer's Disease	107
Chapter 13	The Principle Applied to Diseases of Kidney, Heart, ADHD, Mental Illness and the Human Conciousness	123
Chapter 14	A Medical Tool for Diagnosis and Treatment by Cell Transplants in Order to Restore Damaged Flows	129

Chapter 15	**Two Different Theories Dealing with the Human Body**	137
Conclusion		141
Epilogue		147
Appendix I:	**Reality and the Paradigm of Relations**	151
Appendix II:	**Concepts Understanding Reality, Its Transformations and Its Different Shapes**	163
References		175
Index		177
About the Author		181

Prologue

Living our lives, we normally take our bodies and brains for granted. They just function when we work, study, walk, travel, sleep, eat and make love.

Then, suddenly, my testicle begins to grow, but since I always expect the body to behave well, I ignored it at first. After some months it became difficult to sit normally, since the testicle was rather big, even though it did not hurt and I could do my jogging as usual.

So, I asked a physician what this is.

- It is cancer, testicular cancer, the doctor said.

The answer almost made me faint.

- Now you have two choices, said the doctor. We can do the surgery tomorrow, Friday (it was now Thursday) or on Monday.
- Tomorrow, was my immediate answer.

Then the doctor gave me straight the prognosis.

- If it is seminoma, you will have a 95% chance of survival. If it is teratoma, you will have a 50% chance of survival.

However, it turned out to be seminoma, and I did survive. This was my first time understanding that I had a body and a brain, which might not live for ever.

At the age of 38, I accelerated in living my life, even though I had always been very busy, since I fully understood that I had to live now – fully.

Later on in my life I have survived five more times; AV-block III, and a car accident when my heart stopped. This was due to AV-block III and lack of oxygen to the brain, which made me faint at rather high speed (and those who saw the car with me sitting inside could not possibly believe I survived). Then

I survived blood poisoning and thrombosis, and recently a stroke in the brain stem.

So, living my seventh life, I continue to live fully. Well aware that life will end someday.

However, I have become very interested in the system of the human body. How it functions and what happen every day and every second, how to find the logic behind the amazing body and all its organs and cells and how they are coordinated and of course how to cure and prevent diseases.

I had to give some years of my life to the amazing science of medicine, trying to understand the human body.

Please accept an odd outsider's effort at understanding the human body. In the best case there might be some grain of gold. It is also motivated by trying to find new angles, since there are still unsolved problems within the science of medicine. That's to say, the science of medicine deals with challenging problems, such as:

1. The cause of cancer is not known.
2. The cause of neurodegenerative diseases is not known.
3. Structures at the level of 2-20 nanometre are not concretely known.

It might be difficult to find solutions for diseases as cancer and neurodegenerative diseases if we do not understand the most basic structures within the human body.

Instead of such mechanisms as integrin, ATP synthase, homeostasis and the sodium-potassium pump we need to find an alternative explanation when it comes to the organization of flows of masses in and between systems of the human body.

Even the molecule of DNA gets a new interpretation.

The new concept is TRANSFORMER, i.e., there is interaction between the pathway, its infrastructure and the packages - they are woven and interconnected together.

Packages enter the pathway in order, then by the infrastructure they are organized and transformed into a new shape; a new entity occurs, e.g., cells, organs, humans and species.

It can be summarized like this:

Prologue

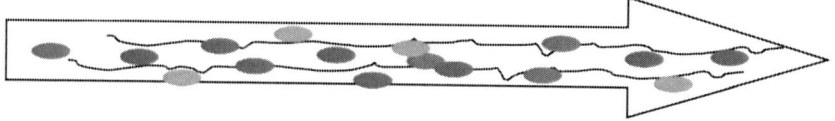

Figure 1. The Transformer of masses.

There are transformers all over reality. DNA is one transformer transforming masses to new cells; Black Holes are transformers transforming masses to new galaxies; Transformers transforms masses to new inorganic shapes, e.g., changes of the Earth.

At this stage it is comforting to quote my favourites and idols:

"To avoid criticism say nothing, do nothing, be nothing."
Aristotle (384 BC – 322 BC)

"Do not fear to be eccentric in opinion, for every opinion now accepted was once eccentric."
Bertrand Russell (1872-1970)

"Every individual ... has to retain his way of thinking if he does not want to get lost in the maze of possibilities. However, nobody is sure of having the right road, me the least."
Albert Einstein, May 25, 1953

"What really make science grow are new ideas, including false ideas."
Karl Popper (1902-1994)

Acknowledgments

Since it is risky to write and think in a new way all on your own, there might occur blind spots, which is normal. Then help from skilled persons will help you to see them.

Three persons have really made this theory more understandable. They are Christian Geisler, Nils-Erik Sturesson and Stig Svensson.

For inspiring and constructive discussion I really want to thank them all.

Google has to be mentioned, since it is an irreplaceable source of information. Most of the material used from Google is well known to all; they mostly belong to every man's general education. I use all material based on fair use and fair dealing, since it is in the best interests of science and that knowledge advances.

Introduction

The theory in this book presents an alternative understanding of the human body based on *one principle* by using the criterion of *simplicity*.
It all starts with *one fundamental postulate*:

Nothing exists in isolation; everything exists in relations.
Then, *one simple principle* derives from the postulate, i.e.:

X = aRb,

Where **X** is inflammation and disease, **a** and **b** are systems and **R** is the relation between them.
Throughout the entire investigation of the human body, e.g., DNA, integrin, ATP synthase, sodium-potassium pump, inflammation, diseases as cancer and neurodegenerative diseases ALS, MS, Alzheimer's and Parkinson's *the principle is followed consistently and consequently*.
As the human body is very complex, consisting of cells, digestive system, molecules and muscles, to mention just a few, a formal principle is of the utmost necessity.
We have now followed guidance from Albert Einstein and Aristotle; trusting Albert Einstein's and Aristotle's cleverness by searching for a principle might be the best starting point.
Albert Einstein: "I came to the conviction that only the discovery of a universal formal principle could lead us to assured results. How, then, could such a universal principle be found?"
According to Aristotle, wisdom is knowledge of principles and causes, and so studying principles and causes is the most fundamental and valuable study in philosophy. Aristotle wrote in the book Physics: "... if we are to gain scientific knowledge of nature as well, we should begin by trying to decide about its principles."

Principles are the base for many ideas within science, politics, and religions and in daily life. Human thinking is based on principles. Most advanced thinking starts and ends with a principle.

How is it possible that different parts of reality and nature are based on separate principles? Can nature have the capacity to let different parts of reality be controlled by different principles?

I believe the answer must be: 'no'. Nature always follows the easiest way of behaving for the reason of simplicity. Then there are no doubts, in all cases of behaviour, about how nature will behave.

The conclusion must then be that there is only *one principle* that guides everything in nature.

This is prime and crucial for the understanding of the human body.

Furthermore, we must focus our search for the principle that it is based on simplicity. Now it seems that basic science is too complex, clunky and tricky. It lacks elegance and simplicity. This is true mostly of the standard model, but also of ATP synthase, integrin and the sodium-potassium pump.

The ultimate goal is to find the simplest principle of the Universe.

So, besides being an important principle, the concept of simplicity has a meaningful role to play, since reality is based on simplicity![1]

There are many theories which are too complicated, such as the standard model based on twenty parameters, which all have to be coordinated, and the ATP synthase model, using questionable and complicated concepts.

Sometimes it is necessary to start all over again, whether it is in science or any other subjects of life.

This is my attempt to understand the human body guided by the rule of simplicity!

Both the molecular machine ATP synthase as well as the sodium-potassium pump and integrin are challenged and questioned, since I do not think they exist and no one has seen them in reality. They are only scientific illusions based on invalid logic. We cannot see them and observe how they behave, since they are all of the size of 20 nanometres (one nanometre is one thousand-millionth of a metre).

I hope to replace them with the phenomenon of a transformer. This part is the tricky one to prove.

---

[1] These giants told us that simplicity is the ultimate whish and desire. Albert Einstein: "Everything should be made as simple as possible, but not simpler." Isaac Newton: "Nature is pleased with simplicity. And nature is no dummy." Leonardo da Vinci: "Simplicity is the ultimate sophistication."

Introduction

A transformer is based on the stipulation that simplicity rules in reality, whether it is the human body, Nature or the Universe.

When masses move in the human body, they pass different organs and their cells. For each pass of a border there is a transformer which directs the masses, which then show up in new shapes, e.g., new molecules, cells and waste.

When we fully understand how masses move and how masses transform in the human body, we are close to treatments for many diseases.

When anything is explained as complicated, including many - too many - factors for its functioning, we have to be suspicious.

There are many examples though the history of science, such as ATP synthase, the sodium-potassium pump and the Standard Model.

Nature and all its content are based on simplicity. Otherwise nature would fail to function.

Furthermore, we maybe need to change perspective, away from the view that physics is the starting point, but to say instead that medicine is the starting point.

The accepted opinion is that physics is the most fundamental science and that chemistry, medicine and other disciplines are built on it.

I am not sure this is the final answer and I will argue that, most likely, the fundament and foundation of science is not based on different matters/materials as in physics, but on the logic of principles, dealing with *the behaviour of objects in all sciences*, i.e., *how the behaviour of (the physical) reality occurs, regardless of its content.*

Once we define the concepts *physical* and *reality* to mean the same thing; i.e., in saying "reality" we are also saying "physical," they are just two concepts denoting the same "thing" - then concepts and postulates dealing with physics do not have implications for other disciplines. An example is the science of medicine, since by this definition medicine deals with reality and might as well be the starting point for all sciences, by launching this new principle – as shown in this book.

Today the science of medicine is mostly based on two postulates:

1. Causal reasoning, i.e., to make sense of cause and effect.
2. The human body is controlled by the laws of physics.

If we stipulate that reality, whether it is the Universe, the Earth, Nature, Society or the Human Body, has one and only one principle which lies behind it all, then we must leave any specialized scientific discipline, since they all have their own principles and theories.

By using the principle X = aRb, where X is inflammation and disease, we find the lowest common denominator of diseases to be damaged or broken R, i.e., damaged flows between a and b.

Consequently cancer and neurodegenerative diseases are not caused by genes, they are caused by damaged aRb, i.e., damaged flows.[2]

In Chapter 1, five main postulates are introduced for reality, including medicine, and then in Chapter 2 and 3 the entire principle takes its appearance, and in the following chapter the theory is applied to established concepts and to different diseases.

As the reader will notice, the authors impatient increases continuously as the chapters passes. So, in the end of the book the impatient culminate. Please excuse me for this, but trust I will come back and make the logic even better.

---

[2] "Literally as well as metaphorically, the man accustomed to inverting lenses has undergone a revolutionary transformation of vision." Page 113; Thomas S. Kuhn: *The Structure of Scientific Revolutions.* 2012.

Chapter 1

Postulates

In this chapter the established postulates of medicine are questioned and new postulates are introduced.

Dealing with reality by science or by common sense, we always have - implicitly or explicitly - postulates guiding our thoughts. We just don't look into reality with an open mind and, mostly, we rely on preconceptions.

That's why the starting point will be to clarify the postulates used. Postulates that the theoretical foundation of medicine rely on, from the point of view of this thesis.

These postulates are not *a priori*, they are *a posteriori*. This means that they are the conclusions after dealing with reality for many years.

1. All consists of the world today, the world of the past and the world of tomorrow.
    1.1 Everything that ever existed, exists or will exist is a part of All.
    1.2. All is dynamic – All is "alive."
    1.3. All = **X.**

2. One world exists today.
    2.1. The world is a part of All.
    2.2. Anything that does not exist today is not part of this world.
    2.3. The world is dynamic – the world is "alive."

3. Any world is differentiated into component parts each one of which stands in relation to another.
    3.1. It all hangs together.
    3.2. Nothing lives in isolation.
    3.3. It all hangs together through a relation - **R.**
        3.3.1. Since it all hangs together; nothing is in isolation.
        3.3.2. The relation is superior to the parts**, a, b, c** …
    3.4. If the relation is superior, there will be no cause and effect between the parts.

3.5. The relation makes the parts' existence possible.
  3.5.1. Without relation the part will die and disappear.
3.6. The concept of relation explains a system.
3.7. All systems are arranged in a logical hierarchy. If a superior system collapses, then all subordinate systems will collapse.
3.8. All systems of relation, at a certain time, constitute the world.
  3.8.1. Everything that happens, happens only one time. Nothing that happens will happen again. The unique disappears and will never come again.
  3.8.2. Everything which is now will be something new.

4. Everything that exists is physically concrete.
  4.1. Meaningful concepts are concretely interrelated.
  4.2. Abstract concepts must be able to be derived from concrete concepts.
  4.3. The sentence expresses the thought in a way which is perceptible for the senses.
  4.4. There are no meaningful concepts without concrete meanings.
  4.5. The contents of thoughts are concrete.
  4.6. That which is concrete either exists or does not at a certain point of time.
  4.7. The combination of article 3 and articles 4.1 – 4.6 is the world alive.

5. Thoughts about concrete facts are meaningful propositions at a certain point of time.

Today, reiterated, the science of medicine is mostly based on two postulates:

1. Causal reasoning, i.e., to make sense of cause and effect.
2. The human body is controlled by the laws of physics.

The new postulate for medicine is:

3. *Nothing exists in isolation; everything exists in relations.*

This postulate is valid for scientific objects as well as for human sciences, i.e., the postulate is at the most fundamental level, before we even think of science and humans; this is valid for all objects and all beings.

However, let us first investigate postulates 1 and 2.

1. When it comes to causal reasoning, i.e., to make sense of cause and effect, we know that the three causes of diseases are injury, toxicity and deficiency. We also know quite well which components causes diseases, e.g., processed food, physical and emotional stress, electromagnetic radiation, lack of calories and water, lack of rest, lack of fresh air, lack of sun and lack of love.
However, how to describe the detailed and concrete chain of occurrences linking these components to the diseases? How and in what way, *concretely*, does a cause generate an effect?
2. The human body is controlled by the laws of physics. Over time we must expect and accept that the laws of physics will be changed, so the science of medicine should not rely too much on them. Physics still has unsolved questions to deal with, e.g., how to unite the theory of general relativity and theories of quantum. So the postulates which rely on physics are not, over time, stable enough to have as prerequisites for medicine. A new paradigm of physics will come, as has always been the case.

Sometimes postulates 1 and 2 are confusing, stating that a force, a causal power, is the cause of an effect, e.g., a disease. Force is a concept used in physics, e.g., a body in rest needs some force to go into motion, and it is a force that causes a unit to change its motion.

Based on statistics, such as Austin Bradford Hill's well-known nine criteria, we identify smoking as the cause and lung cancer its effect. This is a causal relationship, but, again, *how to describe the chain of cause and effect in concrete terms?*

This mechanical view finds nature as a system of causes and effects in space and time. But this view restricts our mind and, since we must look further, it can also damage our thinking. This is understandable, but it will damage our opportunities to understand more of the reality of medicine and the human body.

Let us now turn to postulate 3 and how it might explain diseases and how that would affect medicine as a science.

Chapter 2

The Principle of Relations

The principle is based on three dominant stipulated postulates:

1. Nothing exists in isolation; everything exists in relations.
2. Movement is a property of reality.
3. Every concept has to represent reality directly and concretely.

Now we need to define some important concepts. Then we will have a platform for understanding the human body from a new perspective, even if this is obvious for most physicians, i.e., nothing exists in isolation, not a part, not a system; everything is connected via continuous flows and their impacts between all parts and all systems. Consequently all cells and organs in the human body receive and deliver flows of packages in and out of cells and organs each microsecond; the human body also receives and delivers flows of packages outside of the body, e.g., eating, breathing, working, loving and socializing.

Based on postulate 1, the fundamental concepts and the fundamental equations behind the laws of relations will be the following:

The concept relation relates to reality by showing that there are relations between all parts in reality, where:

1. **a, b, c** ... are any system, subsystem, unit or part in any field of relation in Universe, e.g., suns, planets, moons, galaxies, atoms, molecules, cells, organs and species.
2. The relation, **R,** is a flow (wave) of packages, p_{1-n}, e.g., quarks, protons, neutrons, electrons, photons, proteins, fats, polysaccharides, between a, b, c ... in any field of reality.

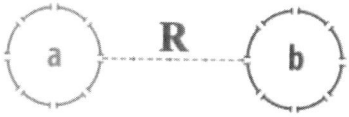

Figure 2. The basic model of relations.

Based on the postulate - *nothing exists in isolation, everything exists in relations* – in combination with 1 and 2 above, the principle is

X = aRb

The principle of relations claims that between all systems and between all parts of any system, S, there is a continuous flow of packages p_{1-n}, i.e., in aRb, $R = p_{1-n}$, and thus the formula is

S = ap_{1-n}b

S is a complex of relations between all parts and elements in the system, i.e., the a, b, and c are complex systems, which send and/or receive flows of packages, i.e., p_{1-n}

$$R = \sum p_{1-n} = p_1 + p_2 + p_3 \ldots p_n$$

The big challenge is now to identify all the *p* in all relations and to identify, certainly and concretely, the logic of

$$S_1 = (a_1 R_1 b_1)\, R_2\, (a_2 R_3 b_2) \ldots$$

The Principle of Relations is based on these statements:

1. There cannot be any fixed atomic facts and elementary propositions.
2. There are no values which are true or false, but only true or false at a certain point of time.
3. Based on the postulates in Chapter 1, the concepts of conjunction, disjunction, implication, negation and plus are not valid. Nature is not based on the logic of conjunction, negation and implication; it is based on the logic of relations.

Based on X = aRb and S = ap_{1-n}b any system is and can be described as complex flows. We might call them wave functions, since a wave function is a flow of masses.

A wave consists of masses which stand in relation with systems. From system *a* the wave of masses moves to system *b*. This is valid for all masses in the Universe, e.g., galaxies, planets, suns, moons, atoms and elementary particles.

We need to find out how the emission and the absorption of these masses of the systems *a* and *b* operate and function. Then gates are crucial and important, and they can schematically be shown as in these two models:

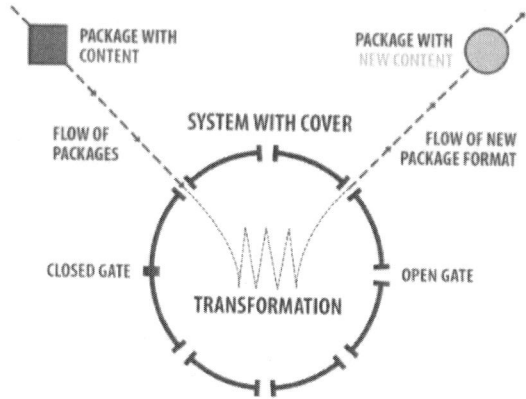

Figure 3. Showing emission and absorption of masses.

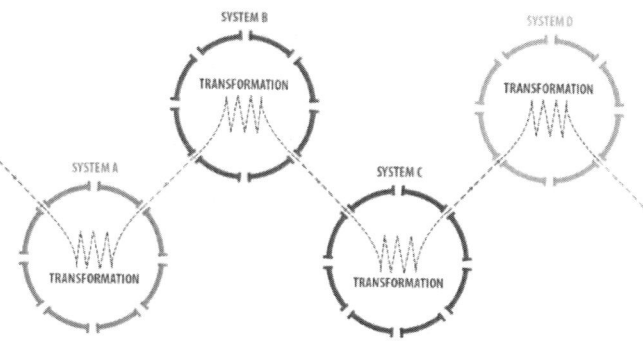

Figure 4. Showing emission and absorption of masses *between* systems.

Then, let us apply these two pictures for the entire Universe, and with our imagination we can understand the complexity, as this model tells us:

The model shows how flows move between parts transporting packages and they must not be taken for gravitation and energy, i.e., these flows are the foundation of reality, out of which gravitation and energy emerge.

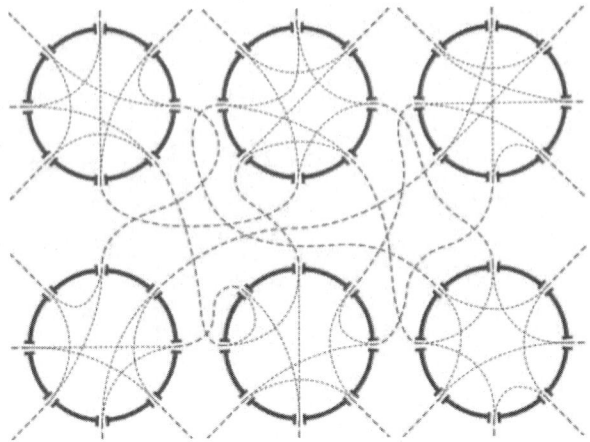

Figure 5. The model of Reality.

Applications of the Principle

X is all and is equal to N, nature, which has all possible contents in the entire universe. The paradigm's equations:

$$S = (aRb)^{-\infty} \tag{1}$$

The system S constitutes of finite relations between a, b, c …

$$R = \sum p_{1-n} = p_1 + p_2 + p_3 \ldots p_n \tag{2}$$

R is the flow of packages, with different content in different systems

$$R_S = (\sum p_{1-n} = p_1 + p_2 + p_3 \ldots p_n)^{\infty} \tag{3}$$

R_S is a system of relations

$$S = (a_{1-n}R_{1-n}\, b_{1-n})R\infty(c_{1-n}R_{1-n}d_{1-n}) \ldots \tag{4}$$

To identify all relations in all systems is a complex work

$$X = S_U R S_E R S_A R S_H R S_B \tag{5}$$

The Principle of Relations

X is the Nature, consisting of relations between the Universe, U, the Earth, E, the Atom, A, the Human, H, and the Brain, B, to mention some systems in Nature.

$$R \to G; \quad R \to m_1 \times m_2/r^2 \text{ and } R \to G\mu\upsilon 8\pi T\mu\upsilon \tag{6}$$

What manifests as gravitation is the flow of packages.

$$R \to E \tag{7}$$

What manifests as energy is the flow of packages.

$$R \to F \tag{8}$$

What manifests as forces is the flow of packages.

$$R \to \Psi(t,x) \tag{9}$$

What manifests as quanta is the flow of packages.

$$R \to L \tag{10}$$

What manifests as light is the flow of packages.

$$N \to SP \text{ and } SP^\infty = (aRb)^\infty \tag{11}$$

What manifests as species, SP, is the flow of packages from Nature, N.

$$S_H = (aRb)^\infty = S_i R_1 S_m R_2 S_c \, R_3 S_l R_4 S_r R_5 S_d R_6 S_u R_7 S_{re} R_8 S_n R_9 S_e \, R_{10} S_s \tag{12}$$

The system of the human body, S_H, is a complex of relations between different parts, e.g., the muscular system, S_m and the nervous system, S_n. Now we can reflect how a molecule or cell can be transplanted to a damaged flow in the body, e.g., an intermodal pathway in the heart and the kidney filtration mechanism, in order to cure AV-block III and repair the filtration mechanism in the kidney, which will be shown later.

We must go all the way from fundamental concepts to concrete parts and facts of reality to fully understand it all.

Usually in science small parts are dealt with, and then within any given and well-defined scientific system. Now we must find out how things and beings hang together, and then we can deal with one part at a time. This is very important, since to limit is to restrict our knowledge. This has to be done again, as it used to be the way of thinking of reality.

Since the Principle of Relations has impacts on our understanding of the entire reality, as a new worldview whether it is philosophy, logic and mathematics, physics, chemistry, biology, medicine or society, an appendix I is available to give an overview: Reality and the Paradigm of Relations[3], and appendix II is available explaining: Concepts understanding reality, its transformations and its different shapes.[4]

---

[3] Thomas Nordström: *Reality and the Paradigm of Relations,* published 2021, Nova Science Publishers, New York.

[4] Thomas Nordström: *Concepts Understanding Reality, Its Transformations and Its Different Shapes* (ijsr.net), 2022.

Chapter 3

The Principle Applied to the Human Body

This is the model of the human body, based on the alternative postulate, *nothing exists in isolation; everything exists in relations:*

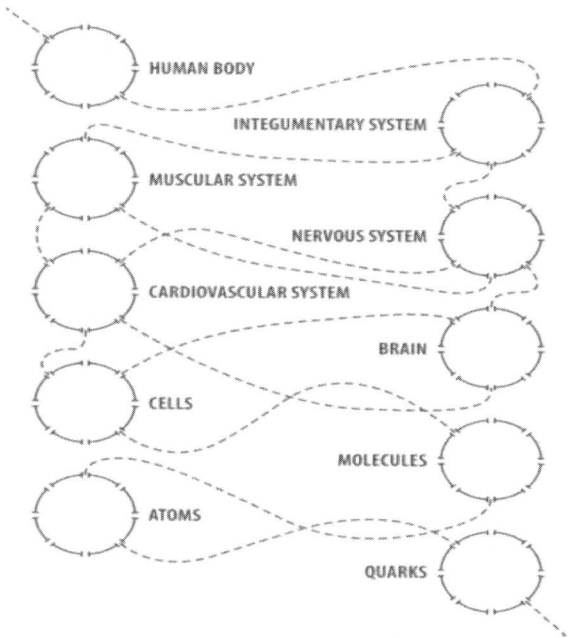

Figure 6. The model of the human body.

The system of the human body consists of flows of packages between different subsystems, i.e., integumentary system, S_i, skeletal system, S_s, muscular system, S_m, nervous system, S_n, endocrine system, S_e, cardiovascular system, S_c, lymphatic system, S_l, respiratory system, S_r, digestive system, S_d, urinary system, S_u and reproductive system, S_{re}.

If S_H stands for the system of the human body, then

$S_H = (aRb)^{-\infty}$ consists of S_i, S_s, S_m, S_c, S_l, S_r, S_d, S_u, S_{re}, S_n and S_e, where each S_{1-11} has its own system of R_{1-10}.

$$S_H = (aRb)^{-\infty} = S_iR_1S_mR_2S_c\ R_3S_lR_4S_rR_5S_dR_6S_uR_7S_{re}R_8S_nR_9S_e\ R_{10}S_s$$

Based on the postulates and the Principle X = aRb, we can look into the System of the Human Body.

With the language of the Principle of Relation we can summarize the system, S, for the human body, H, as

$S_H = (aRb)^{-\infty}$

Since there are 30.000.000.000.000 cells, i.e., 30 trillion cells, where each cell is a living unit, between all cells and organs there are billions and billions of relations, R.

The human body is a complex system of relations between subsystems, down to the smallest elements in and between cells.

The principle is

X = aRb,

where X is any system, including inflammation and disease.

When any R is broken or damaged, i.e., when any flow is damaged, there will be a disorder and disease.

The flow of packages will over time change each of a, b, R and aRb. At t_1 the structure and its contents have one appearance and at t_2 the structure and its contents have another appearance.

When we apply the principle to the human body, the hierarchy of flows can be illustrated as below:

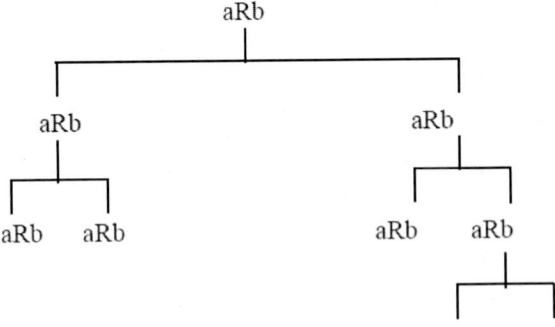

Figure 7. The hierarchy of flows.

The Principle Applied to the Human Body

Now we must identify all a, R and b, which leads us to this table:

$R_1 =$	$a_1 =$	$b_1 =$
$R_2 =$	$a_2 =$	$b_2 =$
$R_3 =$	$a_3 =$	$b_3 =$

And so on for billions of billions of a, b and R within the human body. R contains p_{1-n} and the function of R is as below:

$$R = \sum p_{1-n} = p_1 + p_2 + p_3 \ldots p_n$$

This content will over time change any structure a, b, c in the human body, from the lowest element in the cells to relations between subsystems. Within the body there are a complex R_{1-n}.

Then the hypothesis is that damaged flow dominates causing inflammation, while chronic inflammation causes disease. If damaged flows continue not being repaired, disease will be chronic.

When any R is broken or damaged, there will be disorders and diseases, e.g., cancer, AV-block III, stroke, MS, ALS, Alzheimer's and cardiac infarction.

The Principle of Relations claims that damaged flow dominates causing inflammation, while chronic inflammation causes disease. If damaged flows continue not being repaired, disease will be chronic.

The lowest common denominator for diseases is damaged flow.

Research[5] has clarified how cells shuttle molecules, how vital chemicals are transported within and between cells, how the vesicles contain and release these chemicals and find the right destinations and release the chemical in the right place. Now we have to identify R_{1-10} *between* S_{1-11} and all R_{1-n} *within* all S_{1-11}.

To fully understand the principle there are three crucial factors to deal with:

1. The content of the flow.
2. Transformer's transformation of the content.
3. Structure of masses, e.g., cell, integrin, and DNA.

---

[5] The Nobel Prize in Physiology or Medicine 2013 was awarded jointly to James E. Rothman, Randy W. Schekman and Thomas C. Südhof "for their discoveries of machinery regulating vesicle traffic, a major transport system in our cells."

A Transformer is *the mechanism which directs and leads packages*, e.g., protons, electrons and nutrient molecules, within the cells in the human body.

Now we have to find out how the Transformer works and how it looks. The Transformer is the structure, which organize incoming masses.

Some alternatives:

For each system there are gates, i.e., the transformation mechanism run by the Transformer, whereby the content of the packages is transformed for the next level of the human reality.

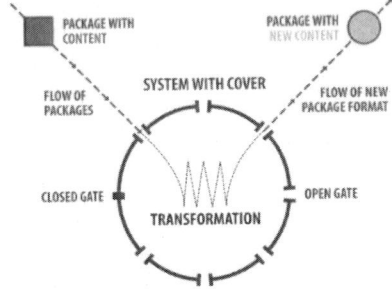

Figure 8. Emission and absorption of masses.

The next image gives an insight into how reality of the human cell works, according to contemporary science:

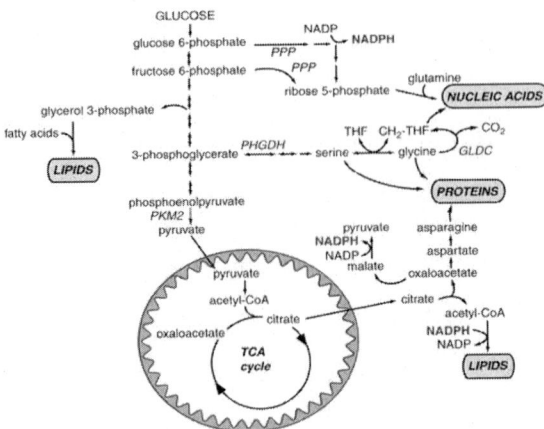

Source: imgurl:https://oncohemakey.com/wp-content/uploads/2017/02/f13-05-97814 55740666.jpg - Bing.

Figure 9. The metabolism of cell growth.

The basic structure of the model of the Transformer, i.e., an alternative explanation, can be presented by the following image:

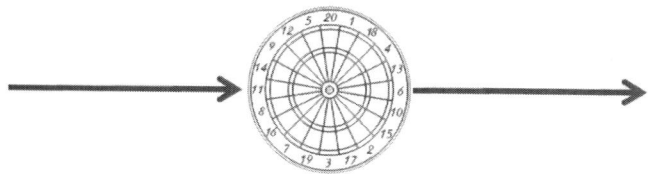

Figure 10. The Transformer.

Throughout reality the Transformer functions by the same principal mechanism, e.g., the Earth, the Sun, the Moon, the Human Body, galaxies, organs and cells in the Human Body.

Since contemporary science relies on the laws of physics and its concepts, then the concept *energy* is found in most explanations of science, e.g., chemistry, biology and medicine.

Then it affects all of the human body, since energy is assumed to be a precondition for survival. Energy is involved in all functions of the human body, such as mental and physical exertions.

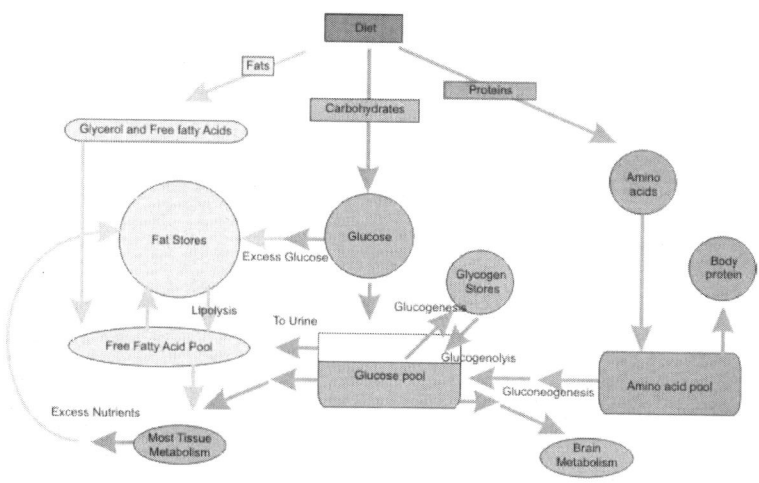

Metabolism Summary
Source: What is Metabolism and How Can I boost It to stay in Shape? - Elana B.

Figure 11. A model of metabolism.

What are the consequences if we abandon the concept energy and instead use the concept of flows of packages, i.e., p_{1-n}?

The conclusion is dramatic, and now the concept Transformer will replace the concepts of ATP synthase and Sodium-Potassium Pump.

Since the flows of molecules of fat, protein and carbohydrates are the most important for the human body, we will now focus these flows.

Above is an image often-used to summarise metabolism to be carefully analysed in this book.

Chapter 4

DNA Transforms Masses

In this chapter DNA is assumed to be an infrastructure building new cells and to function as a *transformer*. This function does not work using the so-called information of DNA, but through the concrete structure of DNA guiding flows of chemical components within molecules. Each set of chemical components takes its position in DNA when their properties fit, via continuous flows.

Since contemporary science claims that DNA contains information, we must find out what information DNA consists of, and what information is needed by all forms of life to function, grow and reproduce.

What is information? Is it a program code or a recipe? By information we normally mean words which describe the concrete level of reality. When a human wants to know how to make a dinner he or she can be informed by a recipe. Building a house, we follow a drawing made by an architect. Manufacturing a car, we follow the design by a computer. Doing heart surgery, the physician follows the instructions of a medical manual. Is the information of DNA a manual of instruction?

What is DNA, really?

DNA, Deoxyribonucleic acid, is a double helix formed by two polynucleotide chains which carries the genetic information intended to affect new cells.

Now we have to find out, in detail, how DNA works affecting the entire human body; and find out in detail, how the so-called information transforms cells.

Does the information have its own affiliation unit? Is there some kind of hard drive storing the information?

There are approximately 300 billion billion combinations within a cell DNA, a number greater than the number of galaxies in the entire universe; based on 300 billion base pairs, that is a number greater than all atoms and subatomic particles in the universe.

So we must ask, is there any computer big enough to handle such an amount of data? No, there are no computers with the storage capacity needed for storing that amount of information.

But, let us suppose that the information is a unit, how does the information reach the molecules consisting of the nitrogen basis A, T, G and C?

How does the information lead to action?

Are there two levels? One level of information and one level of molecules, i.e., one abstract level and one concrete level?

"It is not the chemicals in DNA that store information. Instead it is the ORDER of the chemicals that stores information. These chemicals are the letters of the DNA Instruction Book."[6]

But what does stored information in the ORDER affect?

The Principle of Relations claims that DNA is an infrastructure, i.e., *the mechanism which directs and leads packages of molecules,* to be called transformer, i.e., *DNA is a transformer transforming masses.*

The Principle of Relations claims that the structure of the chemical components A, T, G and C organize how incoming masses are built. At a certain size, the cell has to divide, since it cannot handle too much incoming masses. Then, *genetic information is the physical structure of the chemical components A, T, G and C.* Even if sequences of A, T, G and C can be considered as a four-letter alphabet, they are concrete, solid and coactive chemical components, which allow flows to move in a specific order, guided by the structure. When cells have to divide due to lack of space, new cells occur guided by the structure.

This will solve the problem of storing information, since there exists no information: it is the infrastructure of the chemical components, which automatically organize incoming components.

When flows of components arrive into the structure of DNA, they will follow the pathway within DNA, each taking its position when its properties fit. Flows, consisting of chemical components, arrive and follow the infrastructure finding its place and position.

The model below is one example of the infrastructure of DNA.

This means that we now have two different views of the process for replication: one very fast and one rather slow. Let's call them WC, as in Watson and Crick, and PR, as in the Principle of Relations. Since all processes are made on the smallest level known, i.e., 20 nanometres (nm), it is difficult to fully understand the behaviour of these particles.

---

[6] How Does DNA Store Information? – CreationAndEvolution.org.

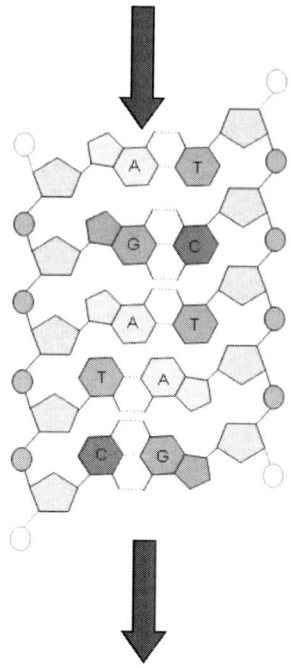

Source: DNA – Wikipedia.

Figure 12. The infrastructure of DNA.

Looking at the X-ray of DNA below we understand.

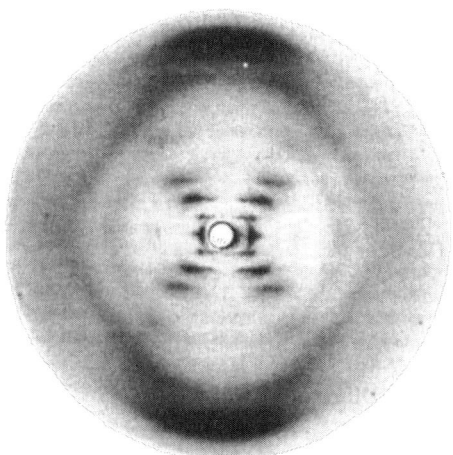

Figure 13. X-ray of DNA.

The X-ray crystallograph shows a crystallized DNA molecule. Source: Franklin's X-Ray Crystallography (mun.ca)

When particles move in DNA, what will it look like? Is it at all possible to find any real picture of DNA telling how it functions? Wherever we may search, we cannot find any pictures, only images made from our guess as to how DNA stores information and how it divides.

The picture below shows DNA under an electron microscope, but does it make us wiser?

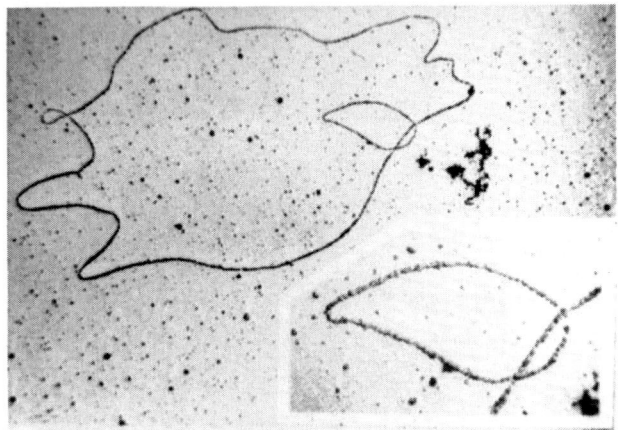

Source: File:DNA Under electron microscope Image 3576B-PH.jpg - Wikimedia Commons.

Figure 14. DNA made by an electron microscope.

Even though science has shown that DNA is a true subject, existing in reality, and science has shown how it behaves, no one has ever seen DNA directly. It is indeed known through indirect proofs and equations, and this can be the phenomenon of Plato's cave. Furthermore, indirect proofs cannot handle the behaviour of reality; they are at best fixed images.

Here we can ask Einstein's question of completeness[7]:

1. "Is the description given by the theory complete?"
2. "Every element of the physical reality must have a counterpart in the physical theory."

---

[7] Page 777 in the PHYSICAL REVIEW, VOLUME 47, MAY 15, 1935: Can Quantum-Mechanical Description of Physical Reality Be Considered Complete? By A. Einstein, B. Podolsky and N. Rosen, *Institute for Advanced Study, Princeton, New Jersey.*

DNA Transforms Masses 21

DNA follows these steps in replication, according to WC, i.e., Watson and Crick:

1. DNA double helix.
2. When hydrogen bonds break the double helix open, the enzyme helicase breaks the helix.
3. Two new identical DNA are produced, each with one new (green) and one old strand (turquoise).

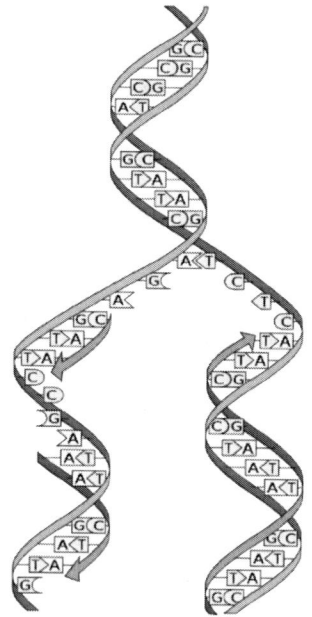

Source: File:Dna-split.png - Wikimedia Commons.

Figure 15. Hydrogen bonds break.

According to PR there are continuous flows in the human body; therefore no hydrogen bonds are needed as well as no enzymes, since the copy has to be made very quickly and performed smoothly and accurately. That means there is no time for chemical reactions, which have been invented by scientists; but we have to understand that nature itself has much more intelligent, smoother and faster solutions. The process is completely automatic.

When new chemical components have filled up DNA, it will automatically break, as a consequence of the size. At this point in time we do not know exactly how this is done.

The molecule of DNA, i.e., $S_{DNA} = (aRb)$, shows the relations between T, G, A and C.

Conclusion

1. Based on the Principle of Relations the theoretical foundation of medicine and DNA will change.
2. Based on the Principle of Relations we have to look at the human body with new eyes.
3. Does mutation occur as an effect of random processes or is it determined? When we use aRb, mutation is determined and not random.

Chapter 5

The Lowest Common Denominator of Diseases

The most important and central frontier in medicine is to find a fundamental principle as the lowest common denominator for diseases, since finding one common cause for most diseases will help the predictability and curing of diseases. It is estimated that over 10.000 diseases exist in the world: a basic principle would ease understanding them.

Based on the Principle of Relations, the hypothesis is that damaged flows dominate causing inflammation, while chronic inflammation causes disease. If damaged flows continue not being repaired, disease will be chronic.

When any R is broken or damaged, there will be disorders and diseases, e.g., cancer, AV-block III, Stroke, Alzheimer's, MS, ALS and cardiac infarction.

Thus, the lowest common denominator for diseases is damaged flows.

Some examples of X = aRb:

1. X = Stroke. When an artery is blocked, the blood supply of oxygen cannot reach the brain's tissues and cells will die, with symptoms such as face drooping and speech difficulties.
2. X = Diplopia, i.e., double vision. When thrombosis in the brain stem damages the flow of blood and draining blood from the brain, visual symptoms such as diplopia will occur.
3. X = AV-block III. When the relation between the SA node, i.e., the sinoatrial node, and the AV node, i.e., the atrioventricular node, is blocked, the pathway has no communication, then AV-block III will occur.
4. X = Heart infarct. When the blood flow in the heart is blocked, lack of oxygen will cause such symptoms as chest pain, shortness of breath and vomiting.
5. X = Cancer. When flows of any network of tubules are damaged, that will cause cancer.
6. X = Testicle cancer. Efferent ducts connect the rete testis and its network of tubules carrying sperm from the seminiferous tubules. Anastomosis connect different parts in the testicle when it is normal.

If the network becomes damaged, i.e., blocked, testicle cancer will occur.

7. X = Neurodegenerative disease, e.g., ALS, MS, Parkinson's and Alzheimer's disease. Now we have to find out if aRb can give some insights into these diseases, i.e., into how damaged flow can be the cause. Can repair of the axonal transport system cure these diseases? How will a change in the anterograde transport affect these diseases? Can the Tau protein repair the damage?
8. X = Alzheimer's Disease. When microtubules are damaged and cannot perform intracellular transport of material, huge amounts of amyloid beta will be crowded outside the cell and neurofibrillary tangles of Tau proteins will occur inside the cell. Can the Tau protein repair the damage?
9. X = Rheumatism. When immune cells cannot find the correct pathway for killing pathogens and instead attack the synovial membrane of joint tissues, i.e., the so-called autoimmunity. Can an antiserum provide a cure?
10. X = Mental illness. The structure of the human psyche, b, is affected by R, from a. When R is damaged, the psyche will develop diseases such as schizophrenia or suicidal behaviour. Isolation and desolation, i.e., damaged R, is often the reason for diseases of the psyche, based on the postulate.
11. X = Suicide. When relations towards other persons are damaged and do not exist, suicide may occur.
12. X = ADHD, Attention-Deficit/Hyperactivity Disorder. It is the society and the relations in the societal network, i.e., the infrastructure, that cause ADHD, via damage in the brain's neurotransmitter system. Flows of packages are essential for normal functioning in any system and when flows of packages of dopamine and norepinephrine in the brain's pathways are damaged, ADHD will occur.
13. X = Schizophrenia. When the pathways of the brain are damaged, it can cause schizophrenia. The damage can result from a situation in childhood, based on contradictory flows of packages.
14. X = Consciousness. Consciousness is the result of the flow of packages which occur from objects outside the human, but it can also occur from objects inside the human, such as body pain and dreams. These packages constitute the memory, which is the consequence of the same molecular movements occurring over and over again, until

there is a pattern in the brain, which will be triggered by the same stimuli of objects. The structure and pattern of the memory is a continuous flow of packages. It will only change by the arrival of new packages, depending on how strongly the pattern has been established. In the worst case, when a mental disorder has come up, it is possible to make the brain healthy again by using an intense flow of alternative packages. Consciousness is then a combination of memory patterns of flows of packages and the flow of packages from outside objects, i.e., consciousness is a flow of thoughts in real time.
15. X = Emotions. When it comes to feelings, emotions and words like love, the content, in concrete concepts, is not that easy to understand. However there is a chemistry of love, where testosterone and oestrogen, dopamine and serotonin are involved, combined with our sense of smell. That is why we need to start at the level of the consequences of a lack of R in these relations.
16. X = Back pain. When muscles are strained, the flow of blood can be damaged, causing pain.
17. X = ...

To be continued ...

Chapter 6

The Scientific Illusion of Homeostasis

In the science of medicine the number of scientists is estimated to be over 200.000 and the total amount of published medical articles yearly is approximately 126,000, i.e., 345 every day and 14 every hour!

Thus, the need for a fundamental principle is truly obvious. It might be the most important and central frontier to deal with in medicine. The situation for the science of medicine looks like not seeing the wood for the trees.

Today two principles dispute, i.e., the principle of homeostasis[8] and the Principle of Relations[9].

In short: The principle of homeostasis argues for stability and the principle of relations argues for change.

These two principles have different views regarding the reasons for disease:

1. The principle of homeostasis finds the reason for disease in lack of homeostasis.
2. The principle of relations finds the reason for disease in damaged flows in and between cells and organs.

According to the principle of relations, the human body is a complex system of relations between subsystems, down to the smallest elements in and between cells.

When any R is broken or damaged, there will be disorders and diseases, e.g., cancer, AV-block III, Alzheimer's and cardiac infarction.

Nature is based on simplicity and continuous flows between a and b, i.e., aRb.

A *Transformer* is *the mechanism which directs and leads packages*, e.g., protons, electrons and nutrient molecules, within the cells in the human body.

---

[8] *The Wisdom of the Body*. New York: W.W. Norton and Company. 1932.
[9] The theory was first published by Cambridge Scholars Publishing: *The Principle of Relations*. 2018. Then the book *Reality and the Paradigm of Relations* was published 2021 by Nova Science Publishers in New York.

Any system has covers. It may just be one cover, but mostly there are many covers within the same system. One cover protects the next layer. There can be many layers in a system, e.g., the human body is entered via hands and mouth - stomach - small intestine – large intestine – kidney – liver – cell; it has its gate and its transformer – mitochondria – chromosome – DNA – gene – ATGC.

The equation behind homeostasis: $ADP + P_i + 3H^+_{out} \rightleftharpoons ATP + H_2O + 3H^+_{in}$ will now change, since it is an unusable and not valid equation, due to the transformer.

Instead, we must find out the components in all chains of flows. Like a train with wagons, then proteins, carbohydrates and fats can show up like this; the commonest components and the most used are these:

… C – H – O – H – N – O – H – C – O – O – H …

Depending on the position and seating, the formula will show up in different shapes. The most common contents are the following:

1. The atoms C – H – O will be present in the flows of fats, e.g., for Cerotic acid $CH_3(CH_2)_{24}COOH$, and for the flows of Carbohydrates, e.g., Sugar $C_{12}H_{22}O_{11}$.
2. The atoms C – H – O – N will also be present in the flows of proteins, e.g., Insulin $C_{257}H_{383}N_{65}O_{77}S_6$, where S stands for Sulphur.

Based on aRb there are no bonds between atoms, there are flows of packages that push and pull the particles together.

Then the formula will be

$S_1 = (a_1R_1b_1) R_2 (a_2R_3b_2)$ …

S_1 is a complexity of relations between all parts and elements in the system, i.e., a, b, and c are complex subsystems, that send and/or receive flows of packages, i.e., p_{1-n}.

The big challenge is now to identify all of p in all relations and to identify, certainly and concretely, the logic of the equation $S_1 = (a_1R_1b_1) R_2 (a_2R_3b_2)$ and illustrated as such:

The Scientific Illusion of Homeostasis 29

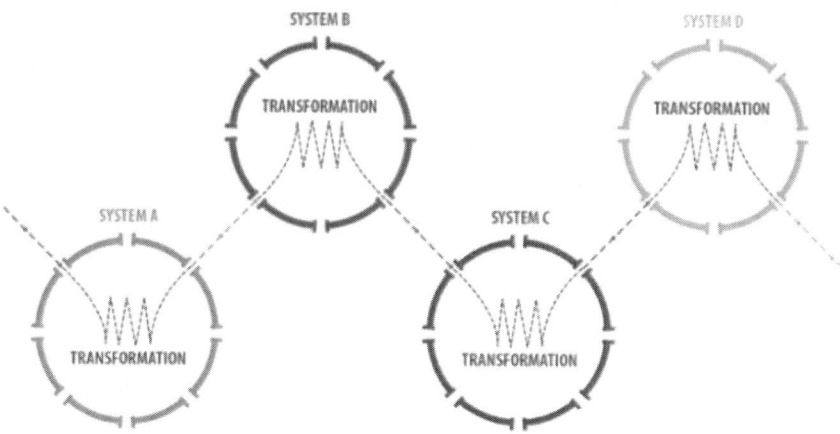

Figure 16. Emission and absorption of masses *between* systems.

The size and volume of any system regulate the flows in and out of the system. When packages leave any system, new packages can enter, i.e., they are needed, since nature abhors vacuum.

How, then, does the Transformer function?

Examining the entire idea of the ATP synthase being a molecular machine must be redone. Taking the Transformer in mind, the conception about ATP synthase may be the most misunderstood part in the human body. When using the concept and phenomenon of a Transformer the conclusion is different.

The cover of any system has a gate where the Transformer is located. When particles get close to the cell, only those particles that fit perfectly can come in. The Transformer can be seen as a paddle wheel, where each paddle can only accept and take one specific particle at a time. The paddle wheel, i.e., the Transformer, takes in one package, particle, after another, e.g., O, H, N, P and C, and out comes a new molecule, e.g., $C_{10}H_{16}N_5O_{13}P_3$.

The shape of a paddle wheel will differ depending on where it is located. Some examples as below might stimulate our imagination (the size will be measured in nanometres, approximately 20-200 nm), where each number can accept only one specific particle from a molecule, e.g., H, N, P, C and O, at the left side, and then a new molecule will occur, e.g., $C_{10}H_{16}N_5O_{13}P_3$, at the right side:

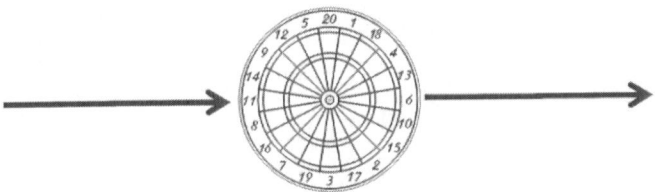

Figure 17. The Transformer.

A Transformer is the mechanism that directs and leads packages, e.g., protons, electrons, photons and nutrient molecules, within the cells of the human body, how new molecules occur and the production of waste.

Complex molecules of glycogen, proteins and triglycerides, change via transformation to simple molecules of glucose, amino acids, glycerol and fatty acids, back to complex molecules as well as waste.

The number of transformers is counted in billions x billions x billions …; they all have the same basic structure but are adapted to fit in. (This goes for all systems in the entire world, e.g., the Universe, the Earth and Nature).

For each system there are gates, i.e., the transformation mechanism run by the Transformer, where the content of the packages is transformed for the next level of reality.

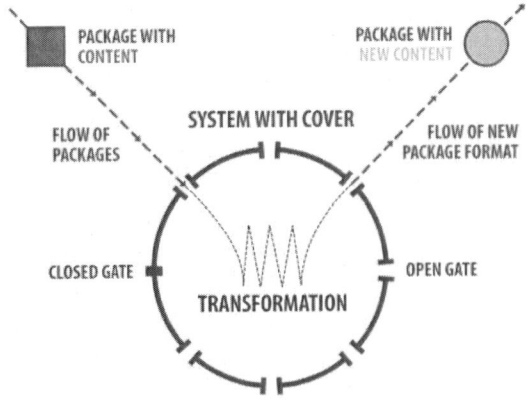

Figure 18. Emission and absorption of masses.

Organs and cells change and diseases occur when R with its packages arrives or not, via the "doors," i.e., the gates, of the cover. There ae chains of transformers, where one after another will transform flows of packages and change the structure for every part of the chain.

Transformers transforms things and beings within the entire reality.

Since the concept and content of transformer is crucial for the principle of relations, this extra explication is needed. But the final view and answer has to be stated.

For now, based on the basic model below, we can imagine how flows are being transformed in the entire Universe.

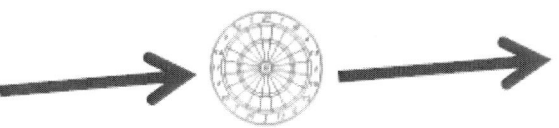

Figure 19. The Transformer of masses.

Imagine you go to the gym. Once inside you follow a scheme made by your PT, personal trainer. After some time your body have, though even minor, changed its shape.

When any mass moves according to a scheme's pathway, e.g., an obstacle course or a cut path, the mass will change its shape.

There is a weave between pathway and packages. Pathway, its flows and its infrastructure constitute a transformer:

1. Packages, i.e., p_{1-n}:

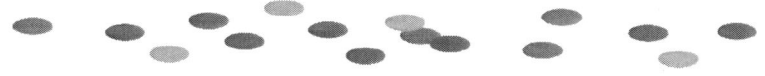

2. Pathway of flow:

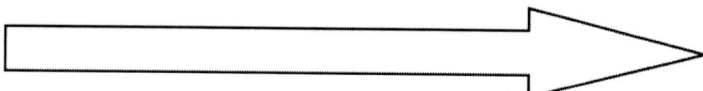

3. Infrastructure:

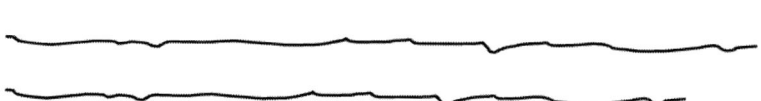

There is interaction between the pathway, its infrastructure and the packages, i.e., they are woven and interconnected together.

Packages enter the pathway in order, then by the infrastructure they are organized and transformed into a new shape; a new entity occurs, e.g., cells, organs, humans, galaxies, planets, trees, stones and water.

It can be summarized like this:

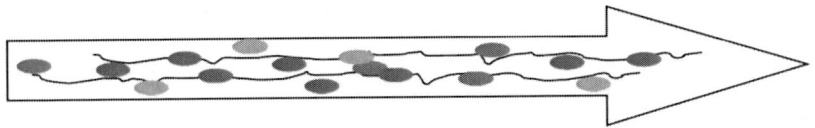

Figure 20. The weave between pathway and packages.

There are transformers all over reality. DNA is one transformer transforming masses to new cells; Black Holes are transformers transforming masses to new galaxies; Transformers transforms masses to new inorganic shapes of entities.

Homeostasis as Concept and Content Has to Be Questioned

The idea of homeostasis, from Greek homoios "similar" and stasis "stable," has a huge impact on the science of medicine. Homeostasis is fundamental to understanding biological systems, including the human body. Its function is to maintain a state of equilibrium within the entire body and its organs. It is a self-regulating process. When an imbalance occurs, it damages any system and disease can occur.

Claude Bernard formulated the phrase *milieu intérieur*, in English *internal environment*. He wrote: "The stability of the internal environment (the *milieu intérieur*) is the condition for the free and independent life"[10].

When Walter Cannon later on introduced the concept homeostasis, that was the underlying principle.

In his book *The Wisdom of the Body*[11], Walter Cannon describes the attributes of homeostasis like this:

---

[10] Bernard, C. (1974) *Lectures on the phenomena common to animals and plants*. Trans Hoff HE, Guillelmin R, Springfield (IL): Charles C Thomas ISBN 978-0-398-02857-2.
[11] *The Wisdom of the Body*. New York: W.W. Norton and Company. 1932. Pages 177-201.

1. "Constancy in an open system that requires mechanisms that act to maintain this system, just like our bodies. (Cannon based this proposition on insights of steady states such as glucose concentrations, body temperature and acid-base balance, authors comments.)
2. Steady-state conditions require that any tendency toward change automatically meets with factors that resist change. An increase in blood sugar results in thirst as the body attempts to dilute the concentration of sugar in the extracellular fluid.
3. The regulating system that determines the homeostatic state consists of many cooperating mechanisms acting simultaneously or successively. Blood sugar is regulated by insulin, glucagon, and other hormones that control its release from the liver or its uptake by the tissues.
4. Homeostasis does not occur by chance, but is the result of organized self-government."

The concept homeostasis has often been illustrated as in the model below:

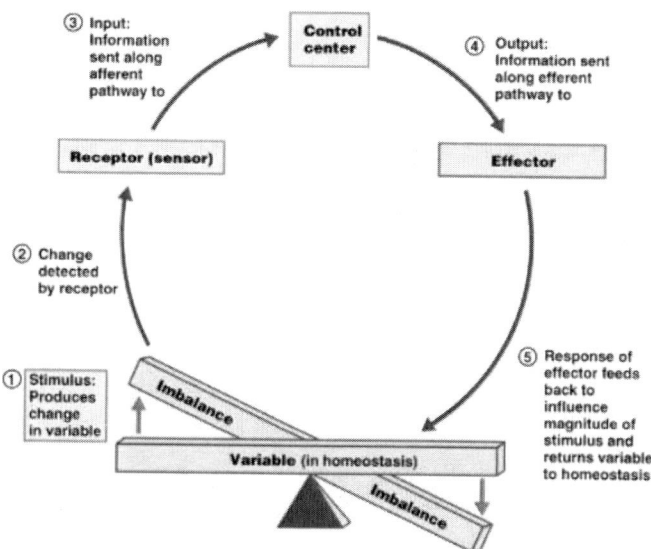

Source: imgurl:https://anatomyandphysiologyi.com/wp-content/uploads/2013/05/Homeostatic-control.jpg - Bing.

Figure 21. Model of homeostasis.

Homeostasis is built on receptor, effector and control centre, but there are also needed such mechanisms as glucose, oxygen, amino acid, fats, endocrine hormones, water, natrium, calcium and enzymes, acting as catalysators making the chemical reaction possible. Then carbon dioxide and ammonia are produced and have left the cell maintaining homeostasis. All these variables need to be controlled to maintain homeostasis. Then, we are told, the internal environment will be regulated.

How, then, we must ask, is control created?

In short, homeostasis means that any biological organism will remain in a steady state, it will be standing still at the same place. However, sometimes the concept dynamic equilibrium is used.

Some common-sense reaction might be that there exists no system, whether in nature or in the human body that over time will be in a steady state maintaining its structure or even its existence. And why does homeostasis not deal with cancer? It is obvious that the concept and the theory of homeostasis cannot be used for understanding the human body or any other system in the entire universe, taking the principle of relations into consideration.

Once we use the concept homeostasis as a fundamental property of biological systems, we are imprisoned in a dead-end. The concept is an obstacle and barrier to a full understanding of how diseases occur and then also of how to find a cure.

Nature, including the human body, is based on simplicity. What happens goes directly without any detours. Then the principle of homeostasis is too complicated to handle the systems within the human body. Each system, such as cells, organs and organelles, has their own function in the entire human body: either they function or they do not. If they do not function it is not caused by a failure of homeostasis, but by damaged flows, which are normally direct and efficient.

Based on the postulate "Every concept has to represent reality directly and concretely," the concept of homeostasis mechanisms cannot be valid. So, we have to look at the concrete level, i.e., aRb and the system of relations, i.e., R_{1-n}.

Even if we now abandon the concept homeostasis, we can use some of its content, but based on the logic of aRb. This applies to such variables as the concentration of CO_2, nutrients, and metabolic end products, pH, and Na^+.

Now, then, the ordering of the variables will follow the line of a flow. A flow which moves seamlessly through any organ and cell.

The so-called regulated variables are blood pressure, blood volume, Na^+ concentration; Ca^{2+}, Mg^{2+}, PO_4^{3-} concentrations; Glucose; Osmolarity; pO_2,

pCO_2, and pH; Temperature. Then, when based on homeostasis, these regulated variables can deviate, more or less. When the deviation is extreme it is called *stress response*, but if it is minor, it is called *defence response*. Under extreme deviations of the variables, the homeostatic mechanisms cannot handle it.

Comparing the two principles "homeostasis" and "relations," the conclusion appears dramatic.

When the principle of homeostasis is used, these variables are regulated by the homeostasis of the cell. But, if we use the principle of relations, it is the status of these variables that make the cell function normally. If the flow of these variables is damaged, the cells functionality will be affected and injured.

In the article[12] "Stress, Inflammation, and Defence of Homeostasis" Raj Chovatiya and Ruslan Medzhitov defend the concept Homeostasis as a fundamental property of biological systems. However, when they define homeostasis of tissues in terms of regulated variables, they open up the possibility of alternative explanations for biological systems.

In some texts we can find the conclusion that even if there is a close connection between inflammatory and stress responses, that relation is somehow *ambiguous;* which gives an indication of difficulties inherent in using the principle of homeostasis to explain disease and inflammation.

So, we have *two opposite views* of the human body, its organs and its cells: *the principle of homeostasis* and *the Principle of Relations*.

Dealing with the causes of diseases, we must now focus on the status of flows within the entire human body and we have to challenge some established concepts, primarily homeostasis, equilibrium and its constant K_{eq}.

Since contemporary science tells that homeostasis and disease have an inversely relationship, then a disease is related to some imbalance in the human body.

Homeostasis means a body in stability and balance or equilibrium. Sometimes dynamics are added, i.e., dynamic homeostasis and dynamic equilibrium. The net movement must be 0, i.e., whatever amount goes in must also go out.

Critical toward this opinion is the direction of the movement, which cannot be reversible.

The reversible reaction, i.e., $\rightleftharpoons$, means equilibrium, i.e., balance and no net change between the components, as explained by the constant K_{eq}.

---

[12] Raj Chovatiya and Ruslan Medzhitov, "Stress, Inflammation, and Defence of Homeostasis," 2014. http://dx.doi.org/10.1016/j.molcel.2014.03.030, in Cell Press. Pages 281-287.

K_{eq} is the equilibrium constant expressing the ratio of products and reactants at equilibrium.

The meaning is that if a system is not at equilibrium, the system itself will direct moves towards equilibrium, quite the opposite of the Principle of Relations.

Equations dealing with ATP synthase in contemporary science view ATP synthase as a catalysed reaction, shown as below:

$$ADP + P_i + 3H^+_{out} \rightleftharpoons ATP + H_2O + 3H^+_{in}$$

ADP consists of $C_{10}H_{15}N_5O_{10}P_2$ and ATP consists of $C_{10}H_{16}N_5O_{13}P_3$.

As we have seen from the Principle of Relations, and the concepts *flow of packages* and *Transformers*, an alternative explanation is possible, i.e., there exists no such thing as homeostasis and equilibrium, since any *flow is one-way only*. Based on the Principle of Relations, neither ATP synthase nor catalysed reaction are needed for understanding the human body. Even the sodium-potassium pump is challenged by the function of transformers.

The body is in a continuous state of movement through flows, where each microsecond and at every moment, the systems of the body are moving, sometimes faster and sometimes slower.

Now, the hypothesis is that the system of flow dominates causing inflammation, while chronic inflammation causes disease.

S_H means the human body system, while HBS means the Human Body Status and is measured by several tests, such as blood pressure, fever, creatinine, glucose, $Na+$, Ca_{2+}, O_2, CRP, EKG and EEG. HBS can also be caused by a malfunction of organs and detection by CT, X-ray and scan (MRI).

Now, the concept Homeostasis will be replaced by the concept Human Body Status, HBS, for two reasons:

1. The idea and principle of Homeostasis is not valid.
2. HBS is based on objective facts.

By restructuring the content of the article "Stress, Inflammation, and Defence of Homeostasis," we will find a new perspective, since now we will use new glasses for looking at the reality of the human body. The glasses are called The Principle of Relations, based on the formula $X = aRb$, where X is inflammation and disease as well as HBS, i.e., the human body status.

The human body is complex, but not complicated. Once we find the basic principle and the theory that underlies the functionality of the human body, we will make it simple to understand the human body.

At this stage the concept of "homeostasis" is replaced by the concepts "system of flow."

If we now also replace some part of the concept homeostasis with the concept functioning, as functioning organs and organisms, we can identify when an organism and its organs are not functioning by making different measurements and tests: blood tests, x-rays, ultrasonography, urine tests, DNA-tests and other observations.

Then we start understanding the human body from objective facts, such as high blood pressure, pain and fever. Blood tests tell us the status of Haemoglobin, Glucose, Cholesterol, Creatinine, Sodium, C-reactive protein (CRP) and many others.

Conclusion

The Principle of Relations replaces the Principle of Homeostasis.

Then the hypothesis is that the system of flow dominates causing inflammation, while chronic inflammation causes disease. If damaged flows continue not being repaired, disease will be chronic.

Instead of finding the reason for disease in lack of homeostasis, we will find the reason for disease in damaged flows in and between cells and organs.

Chapter 7

How Mass Moves in the Human Body

In this chapter we focus how masses move in the human body and how they are transformed.

Today basic sciences have turned into over 633 different sciences and it has been an exponential development over the last century. Almost any field of study has a name, ending with "-ology" from the Greek word logos, meaning ground or reason, such as cardiology for the study of the heart, sociology for the study of society, carpology for the study of fruit and entomology as the study of insects to mention four out of the 633.

Now the need for a fundamental principle of medicine is truly obvious. It might be the most important and central frontier to deal with in medicine. The situation for the science of medicine looks like not seeing the forest for the trees.

Today two principles dispute, i.e., the principle of homeostasis and the Principle of Relations.

The principle of homeostasis argues for stability and the principle of relations argues for change.

Where in reality can we find any system or subsystem, whether within nature, the entire Universe or the human body, which will remain stable over time?

Nowhere of course.

Then it is not decent and applicable to use some principle which is based on stability, stable and similar, i.e., homeostasis.

Nature is based on simplicity and continuous flows between a and b, i.e., aRb.

Instead of finding the reason for disease in lack of homeostasis, we will find damaged flows in and between cells and organs as the reason for disease.

How, then, concretely, does a blockage of flow cause the occurrence of inflammation leading to a disease?

The Principle of Relations and Its Consequences

We can identify, at least four levels in the human body, and each level has a basic structure in common with the others:

1. The human body as a whole.
2. Organs, such as heart, kidney and lungs.
3. Cells and their organelles.
4. The structure of DNA.

The organs of the human body can be shown as two simple overviews, (see below); but they give us the possibility of using our fantasy when it comes to understanding how and which relations exist:

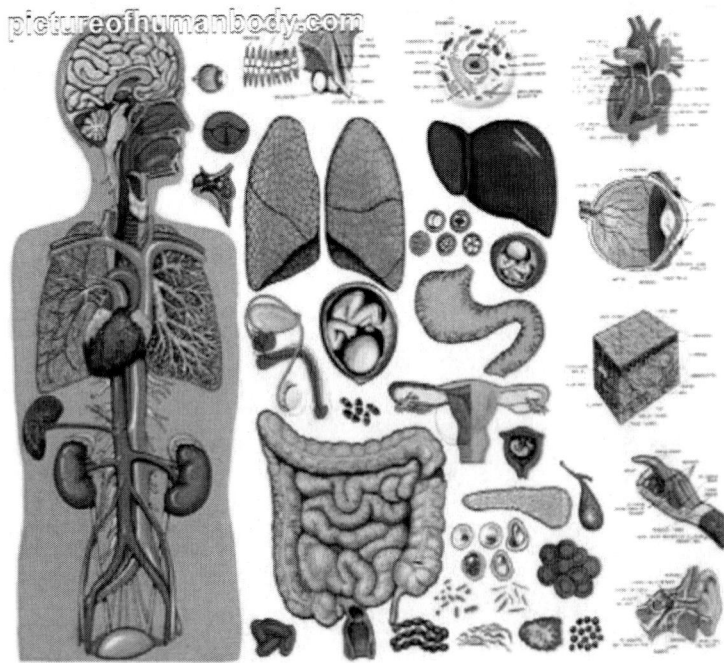

Source: Funny Pictures Gallery: Organs, internal organs diagram, body organs location, body organs, organ (funny-pic24.blogspot.com).

Figure 22. Organs of the human body.

How Mass Moves in the Human Body 41

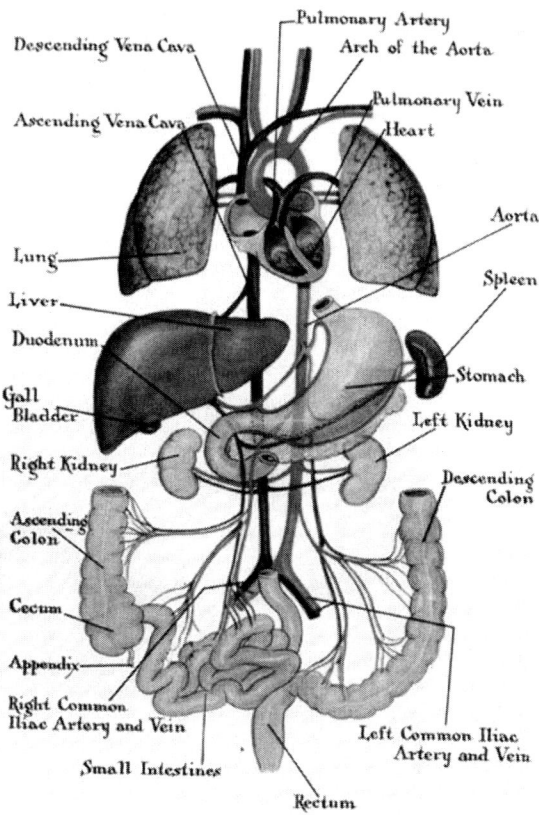

Source: organs+(1).gif (450×664) (bp.blogspot.com).

Figure 23. Structure of the human body.

How can a cell manage all subsystems, the organelles, within its border, the ATP synthase, the sodium-potassium pump, the mitochondria and the DNA?

Since the structure of a cell by its organelles has a similarity with the organs in the body, we can find the common model for both, by using the formula $S_H = (aRb)^{-\infty}$ for the cell C, then the formula will be $S_C = (aRb)^{-\infty}$

Now, based on the Principle of Relations, we have to identify all relations on all levels of the cell. This is crucial for understanding the cell. The most complicated part is how different levels are connected within the cell.

The human body has 30.000.000.000.000 cells. The functionality of a cell is not possible if it is too complicated - the cell must be based on simplicity, i.e., the cell might be complex, but it is not complicated.

The cell, as we are told today, has this structure:

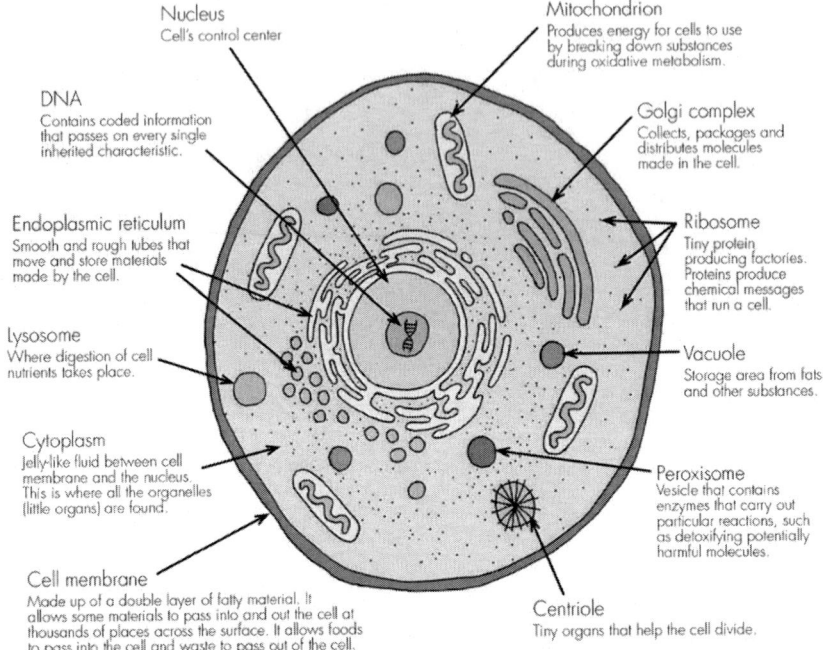

Source: Cells - Haleo.

Figure 24. The cell.

Within the cell, the speed of flows must be high, without any obstacles or blocks, since it all has to run workably and with high agility. Contemporary science tells us that the cell works by letting enzymes carry out chemical reactions. Enzymes break down glucose as well as creating new enzymes and making the cell reproduce. We will call this the hypothesis no 2, as below. Is it possible for these enzymes to be as efficient as is needed in the cells flows?

Flows in the Cell

Based on aRb, i.e., the Principle of Relations, we must find all flows in the cell and how they are connected with each other, starting from molecules passing the membrane until new cells are produced as well as waste. Besides the flows, there are structures, such as chromatin structures, which hold packages of DNA. How these structures of DNA and chromatin are affected by flows within the cell, is one key point.

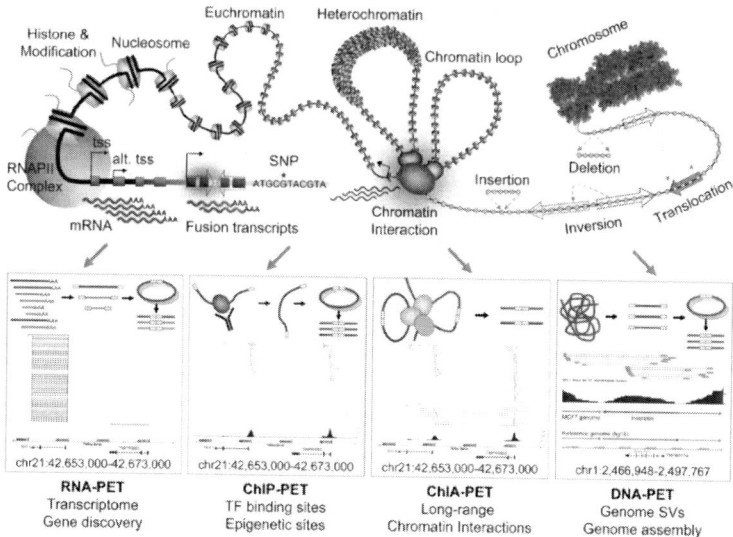

Source: F3.large.jpg (1280×905) (cshlp.org).

Figure 25. DNA from different views.

Does mutation occur as a random effect or is it determined? When we use aRb, mutation is determined and not random. The molecule of DNA, i.e., S_{DNA} = (aRb), which shows the relations between T, G, A and C:

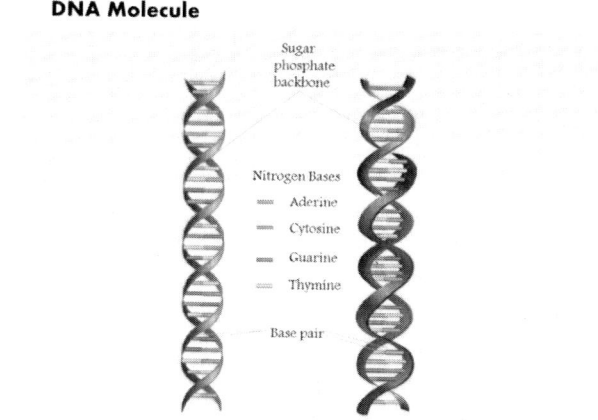

Source: imgurl:https://www.slideteam.net/media/catalog/product/cache/1280x720/ 0/8/0814_dna_molecule_medical_images_for_powerpoint_Slide01.jpg-Bing.

Figure 26. DNAs content.

This next picture made in an electron microscope gives us the impression of a flow:

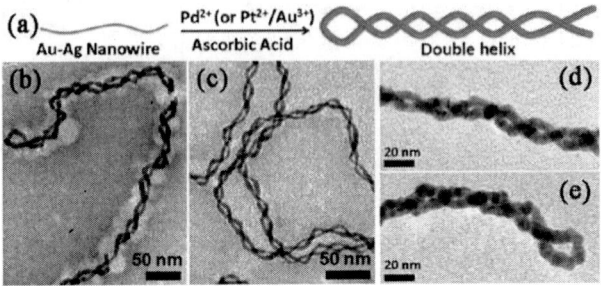

Source: Pinterest.

Figure 27. Electron view of DNA.

What Is Genetic Information?

It is the structure of the chemical components A, T, G and C. Even if sequences of A, T, G and C can be considered as a four-letter alphabet, it is a set of concrete, solid and coactive chemical components, which allow flows to move in a specific order, guided by the structure. Then new cells occur guided by the structure.

The molecule of DNA, consisting of the acronym ACGT, i.e., adenine, cytosine, guanine and thymine, is often shown as this model:

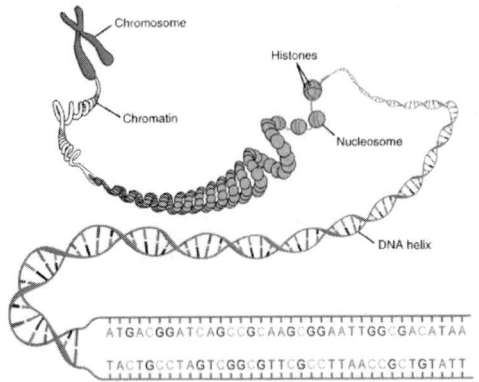

Source: imgurl:http://oerpub.github.io/epubjs-demo-book/resources/0321_DNA_Macrostructure.jpg - Bing.

Figure 28. DNA within the chromosome.

How Mass Moves in the Human Body 45

The DNA molecule consists of two strands, weaved around each other. It is adenine and thymine that make a pair and guanine and cytosine that make a pair. Then it is pairs of AT and CG making up DNA. Then, contemporary science uses hydrogen bonds to make the molecules A, T, G and C hang together, as this model shows:

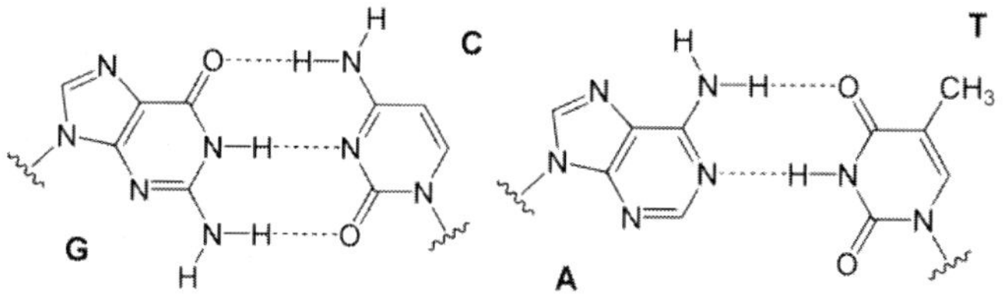

Figure 26. Hydrogen bonds in DNA.

Looking at this model with the eyes of aRb, questions occur:

1. What is the alternative to hydrogen bonds?
2. What in the wall of the molecule can arrange the structure of the molecule?
3. How does a new molecule occur?
4. How do new cells occur?

The Transformer – Reiteration Needed to Understand Enzymes

A Transformer is *the mechanism which directs and leads packages*, e.g., protons, electrons and nutrient molecules, within the cells in the human body, as is to be shown again in this section.

Throughout reality the same principle applies to the mechanisms of a Transformers functions, e.g., the Earth, the Sun, the Moon, the human body, galaxies, organs and cells in the Human Body.

Any system has covers. It can be just one cover, but mostly there are many covers within the same system. One cover protects the next layer. There can be many layers in a system, e.g., the human body is entered via hands and mouth – stomach – small intestine – large intestine – kidney – liver – cell; it has its gate and its transformer – mitochondria – chromosome – DNA – gene – ATGC.

ATP synthase is one transformer which functions in membranes, i.e., the thylakoid membrane and the inner mitochondrial membrane.

Since ATP synthase is an enzyme protein, we can expect that all enzymes are transformers.

In the cover, e.g., the membrane of a cell or the crust of the Earth, there are Transformers. Flows are *directed* via the Transformer into the systems and different subsystems, and so on for all systems and subsystems.

The equation $ADP + P_i + 3H^+_{out} \rightleftharpoons ATP + H_2O + 3H^+_{in}$ will now change, since it is an unusable and not valid equation.

Instead, we must find out the components in all chains of flows. Like a train with wagons, as we may first imagine them, proteins, carbohydrates and fats can show up like this; the most common components and the most used are these:

$$... C - H - O - H - N - O - H - C - O - O - H ...$$

Depending on the position and placement, the formula will show up in different shapes. The most common contents are the following:

1. The atoms C – H – O will be present in the flows of fats, e.g., for Cerotic acid $CH_3(CH_2)_{24}COOH$, and for the flows of Carbohydrates, e.g., Sugar $C_{12}H_{22}O_{11}$.
2. The atoms C – H – O – N will also be present in the flows of proteins, e.g., Insulin $C_{257}H_{383}N_{65}O_{77}S_6$, where S stands for Sulphur.

Based on aRb there are no bonds between atoms, there are flows of packages that push and pull the particles together.

Then the formula will be

$$S_1 = (a_1R_1b_1)\ R_2\ (a_2R_3b_2)\ ...$$

S_1 is a complex of relations between all parts and elements in the system, i.e., a, b, and c are complex subsystems, that send and/or receive flows of packages, i.e., p_{1-n}.

Then

$$R = \sum p_{1-n} = p_1 + p_2 + p_3 ... p_n$$

The big challenge is now to identify all the *p* in all relations and to identify, certainly and concretely, the logic of

$S_1 = (a_1R_1b_1)\ R_2\ (a_2R_3b_2)\ ...$

The equation for this may be illustrated as such:

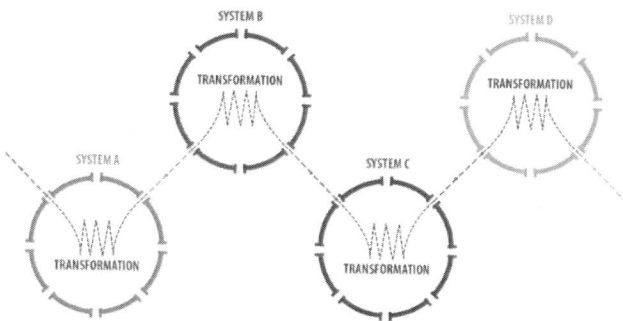

Figure 29. Transformation in different systems.

The size and volume of any system regulate the flows in and out of any system. When packages leave any system, new packages can come in, i.e., they are needed.

How, then, does the Transformer function?

The entire idea of the ATP synthase being a molecular machine must be re-examined and re-worked. Having the Transformer in mind, the conception about ATP synthase may be the most misunderstood part in the human body. When using the concept and phenomenon of a Transformer the conclusion is different. In the following I will explore this path and establish the groundwork for seeing the ATP synthase in relation to the Transformer.

The cover of any system has a gate where the Transformer is located. When particles get close to the cell, only those particles that fit perfectly can come in. The Transformer can be seen as a paddle wheel, where each paddle can only accept and take one specific particle at a time. The paddle wheel, i.e., Transformer, takes in one package, particle, after another, e.g., O, H, N, P and C, and out comes a new molecule, e.g., ATP: $C_{10}H_{16}N_5O_{13}P_3$.

The shape of a paddle wheel will differ depending on where it is located. Some examples as below might stimulate our imagination (the size will be measured in nanometres, approximately 50-200 nm), where each number can accept only one specific particle from a molecule, e.g., H, N, P, C and O, at the left side, and then a new molecule will occur, e.g., $C_{10}H_{16}N_5O_{13}P_3$, at the right side:

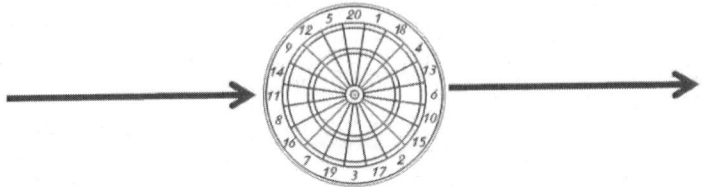

Figure 30. The Transformer.

Let us use our imagination again.

The molecule of a D-glucose chain as below can be seen as a flow of packages, which is directed by the Transformer:

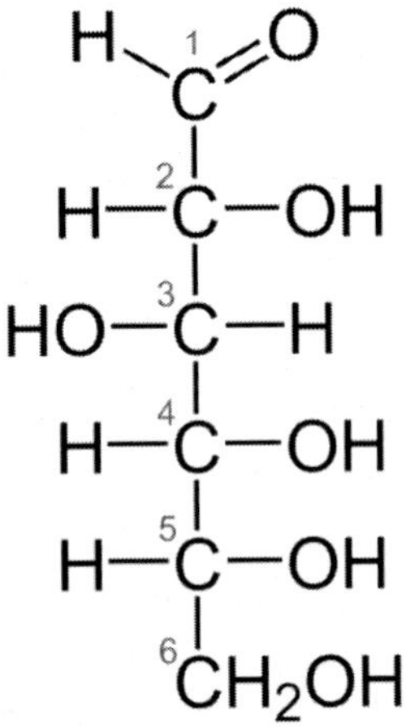

$$\begin{array}{c}
\overset{1}{C}\!\!\begin{array}{c}\diagup\!\!\!O\\[-2pt]\diagdown\!\!\!H\end{array}\\
H-\overset{2}{C}-OH\\
HO-\overset{3}{C}-H\\
H-\overset{4}{C}-OH\\
H-\overset{5}{C}-OH\\
\overset{6}{C}H_2OH
\end{array}$$

Figure 31. The molecule of a D-glucose.

Enzyme as Concept and Content Has to Be Questioned

Contemporary science argues that enzymes are biocatalysts accelerating chemical reactions and converting the so-called substrates to molecules. In metabolic pathways enzymes are needed at each step, in order to reach rates fast enough for sustaining life.

Enzymes consist of chains of amino acids. They are said to be held together by peptide bonds, but even this has to be questioned.

Instead, metabolism is a number of transformations of food made by transformers.

As it seems metabolism in cells is complex, consisting of thousands of genes and proteins. These molecules involve biochemical networks in reactions. How can we understand all of it?

Starting with some basic models we can, step by step, build up and construct an understanding.

Are enzymes transformers then?

The Difference between Enzymes and Transformers

In 1894 Emil Fischer proposed his lock-and-key model dealing with how enzymes function. In 1958 the Induced Fit model of enzyme activity was proposed by Daniel Koshland. The model tried to explain how the enzyme moulds itself to be the same as the geometry of the molecule, once a contact with the substrate came about.

The model below gives some understanding.

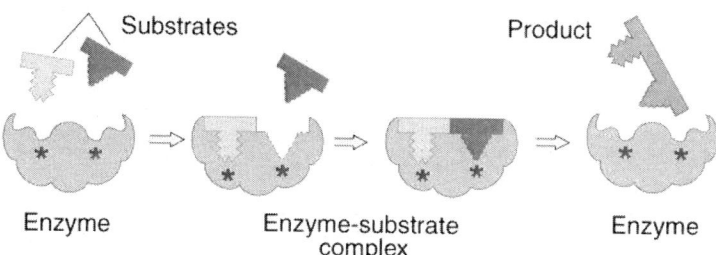

Source: imgurl:https://www.mun.ca/biology/scarr/F09-20bsmc.jpg - Bing.

Figure 32. The induced fit model of enzyme.

The equation below was written by Daniel E. Koshland in his paper, *Application of a Theory of Enzyme to Protein Synthesis*:

^+H_3N --- $CHRCOO^-$ + $H_3N+CHR^-COO^-$ → H_3N^+---$CHRCO$---$NHCOO^-$ +H_2O

This reaction, according to Koshland, requires energy, which will come from ATP, i.e., adenosine triphosphate. This reaction also needs catalysis, since it is too slow. In the process of making protein synthesis, peptide bonds have to be used. It is all done in laboratories with the help of a chemical template, which will control all reactions and fabricate the product.

The understanding of how protein synthesis is generated has not got a complete answer, as Daniel E. Koshland told us in his paper.

In short, the Transformer again:

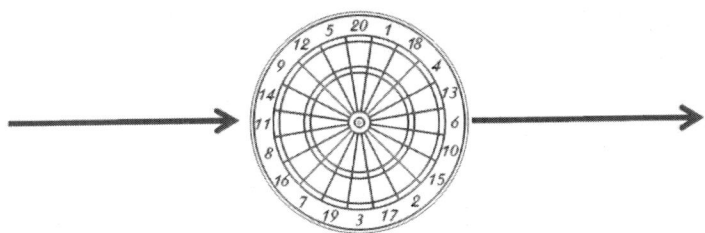

Figure 33. The Transformer.

The Transformer is a complete model, dealing with all flows in the body, by not using homeostasis, ATP synthase, chemical bonding or catalysts.

So far, what is the difference between the two models, the Induced Fit model and the Transformer model? In the table below we start up the comparison:

Property	Model Induced Fit	Transformer
Catalyst	Yes	No
ATP	Yes	No
Bonding	Yes	No
Homeostasis	Yes	No
Position fit*	Yes	Yes
* An individual position in the protein is occupied by one and only one amino acid		

Some Steps Deeper and Further

First, the overall metabolic map, as below.

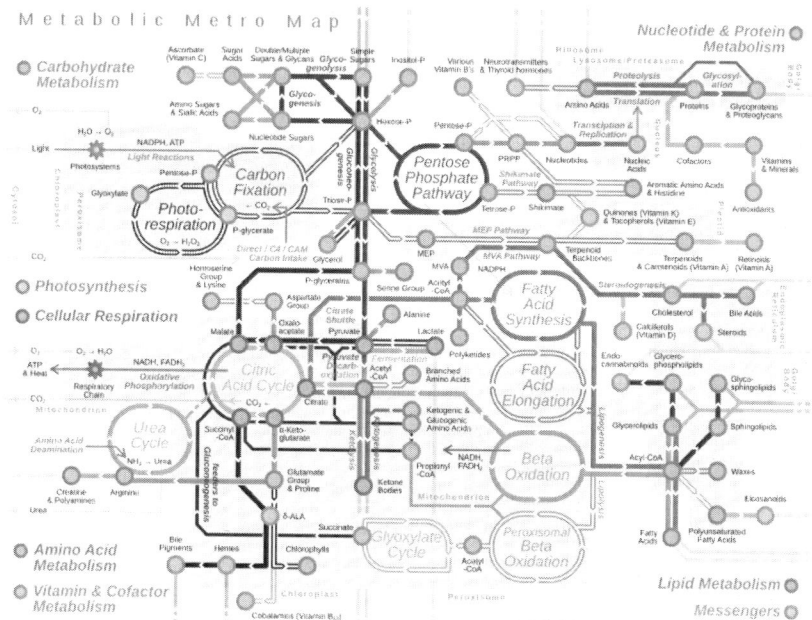

Source: File:Metabolic Metro Map.svg - Wikipedia.

Figure 34. Metabolic map.

Orange nodes are carbohydrate metabolism, violet nodes are photosynthesis, red nodes are cellular respiration, pink nodes are cell signalling, blue nodes are amino acid metabolism, grey nodes are vitamin, brown nodes are nucleotide and protein metabolism, green nodes are lipid metabolism. (When looking at this overview of metabolism in Wikipedia one might click any text to find articles).

Are enzymes transformers and what is a transformer?

The metabolic pathway of glycolysis uses different enzymes, i.e., transformers, to perform the transformation of glycolysis to the molecular pyruvate. Different enzymes, in all eleven, perform chemical modification.

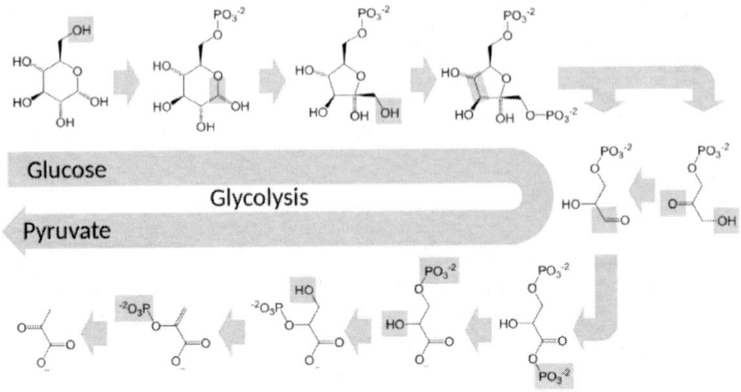

Source: Pinterest.

Figure 35. Metabolic pathway of glycolysis.

The formula of the molecular pyruvate is $C_3H_4O_3$ and via transformation from the molecular glucose with the formula $C_6H_{12}O_6$ and enzymes, i.e., transformers, (red in the figure), the molecular pyruvate occurs and is created. ATP has to be dealt with, since it might be an illusion. This model gives some idea of what happens:

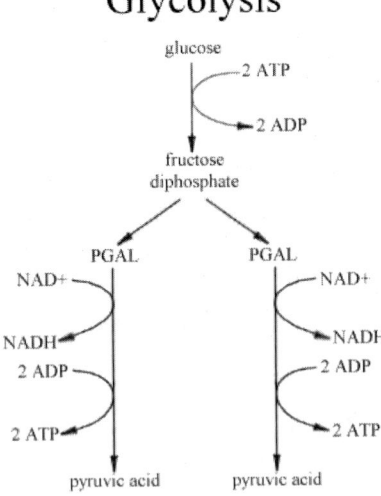

Source: imgurl:https://www.excellup.com/InterBiology/elevenbioimage/11_Biology _14_PlantRespiration2.png - Bing.

Figure 36. The process of enzymes.

The Nobel Prize in Chemistry 2021 takes one step toward reducing the role of enzymes to act as catalysts, by introducing organic catalysts. The press release says this:

> "Organic catalysts have a stable framework of carbon atoms, to which more active chemical groups can attach. These often contain common elements such as oxygen, nitrogen, sulphur or phosphorus. This means that these catalysts are both environmentally friendly and cheap to produce. The rapid expansion in the use of organic catalysts is primarily due to their ability to drive asymmetric catalysis. When molecules are being built, situations often occur where two different molecules can form, which – just like our hands – are each other's mirror image. Chemists will often only want one of these, particularly when producing pharmaceuticals."

The pictures below show this:

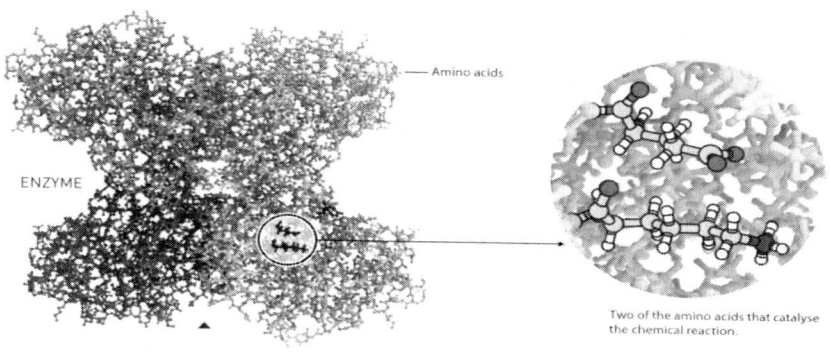

Figure 37. Catalyse reaction.

The next step is to find out how a transformer will reduce both enzymes and organic catalysts to zero, since they are not needed in the flows of the human body.

A Transformer is the mechanism that directs and leads packages, e.g., protons, electrons, photons and nutrient molecules, within the cells in the human body, governing how new molecules occur and waste is produced. Complex molecules of glycogen, proteins and triglycerides, change via transformation into simple molecules of glucose, amino acids, glycerol and fatty acids, and back to complex molecules as well as waste.

The number of transformers is counted in billions x billions x billions …; they all have the same basic structure but are adapted to fit in. (This goes for all systems in the entire world, e.g., the Universe, the Earth and Nature).

For each system there are gates, i.e., the transformation mechanism run by the Transformer, where the content of the packages is transformed for the next level of reality.

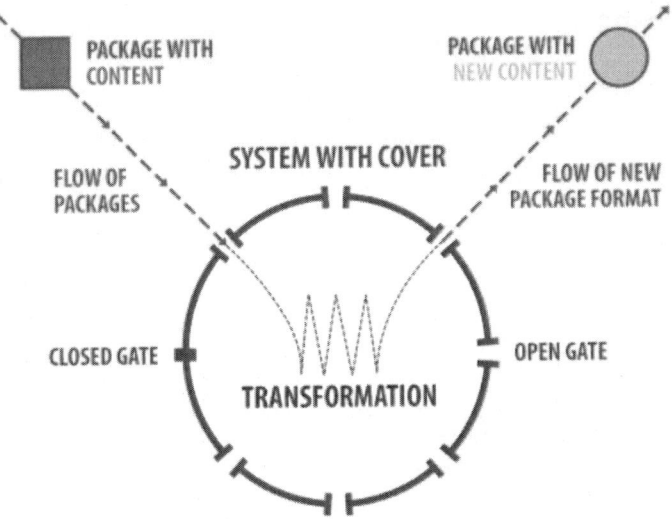

Figure 38. Transformation of packages.

Organs and cells change and diseases occur when R with its packages arrives or not via the "doors," i.e., the gates, of the cover.

The Transformer can be seen as a paddle wheel, where each paddle can only accept and take one specific particle at a time. The paddle wheel, i.e., Transformer, takes in one package, particle, after another, e.g., O, H, N, P and C, and out comes a new molecule, e.g., ATP: $C_{10}H_{16}N_5O_{13}P_3$.

It has to be reiterated: the shape of a paddle wheel will differ depending on where it is located. Some examples as below might stimulate our imagination (the size will be measured in nanometres, approximately 50-200 nm), where each number can accept only one specific particle from a molecule, e.g., H, N, P, C and O, at the left side, and then a new molecule will occur, e.g., $C_{10}H_{16}N_5O_{13}P_3$, at the right side:

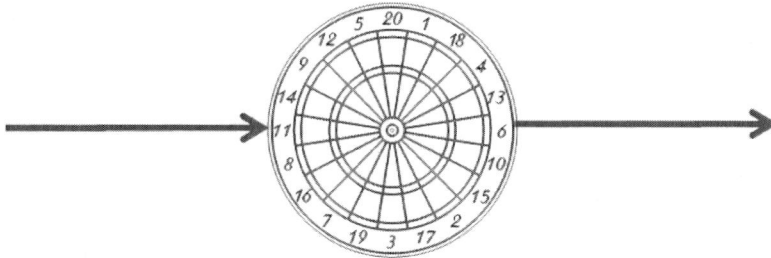

Figure 39. The Transformer.

There will be chains of transformers, where one after another will transform flows of packages and change the structure for every part of the chain. Symbolically it can be shown like this:

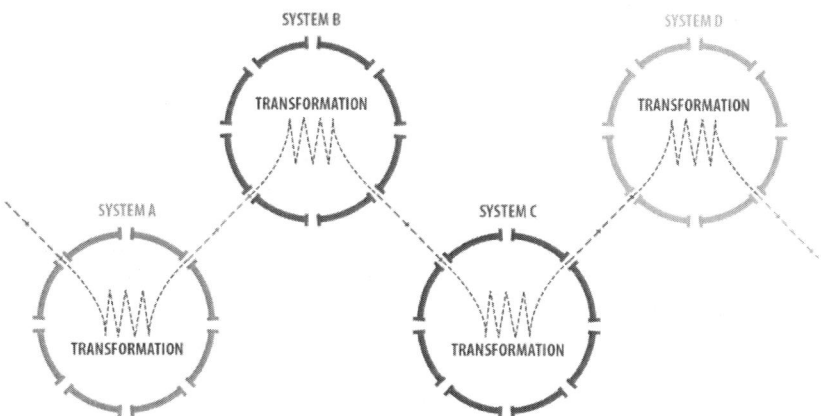

Figure 40. Transformation in different systems.

This model is, like most models made by men, oversimplified. The real structure and function of transformations via transformers, must be reviewed over and over again.

In contemporary science enzymes are viewed as acting as biocatalysts. But they look like transformers, since they convert substrates into new molecules, called products. The well-known image below shows this.

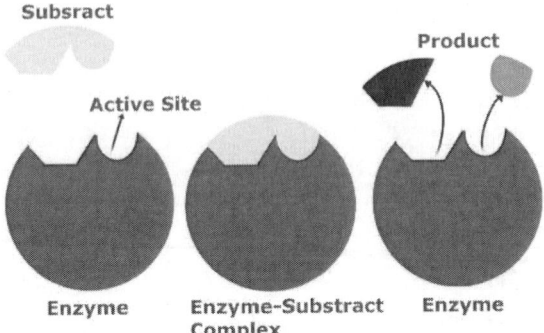

Source: imgurl:https://ibiologia.com/wp-content/uploads/2019/07/enzyme.jpg - Bing.

Figure 41. Biocatalysts.

There are some similarities between these two images (Figures 38 & 39). The next image below is one attempt to understand how the Transformer acts.

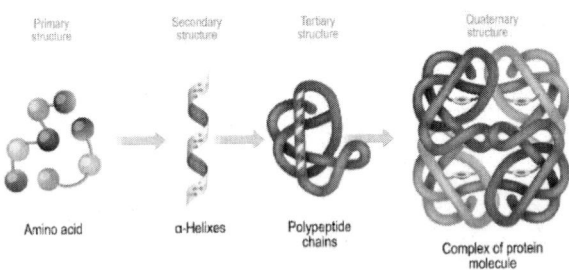

Source: imgurl:https://martinswellness.com/media/wysiwyg/blog/protein-structure-1920x1200px.jpg - Bing.

Figure 42. The transformation processes.

The first possible answer dealing with the physical appearance might be that a transformer is like a floating fluid with properties to handle the transformation of incoming complex molecules to simple molecules and back to complex molecules.

The tricky part is now to understand in detail how this function. The next image gives an idea of how simple molecules are transformed into the so-called secondary structure, and via the tertiary structure create a complex molecule.

How Mass Moves in the Human Body 57

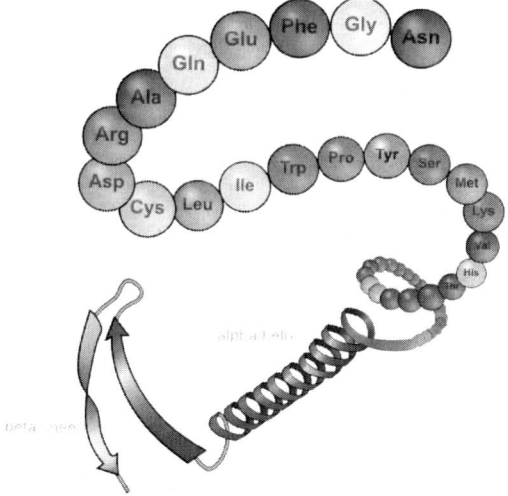

Source: imgurl:https://1.bp.blogspot.com/-5Z-hND0LbKg/XwnsvlUHg9I/AAAA
AAAAOyw/yx9C530JeEwChTBujqG6GqkUajhaZTVaACLcBGAsYHQ/s1600
/1.jpg - Bing.

Figure 43. The process of transformation.

The human body has approximately 30 trillion cells, i.e., 30.000.000.000.000. Then the cell must have some simple functionality or the human body will be a disaster.

Now, we have to understand how the Transformer functions based on the new definition of the concept energy.

So far, energy is involved in the metabolic processes of catabolism and anabolism, often shown in images as below:

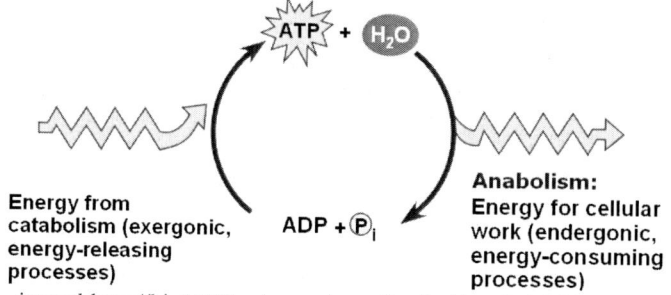

Source: imgurl:http://biol151b.nicerweb.net/Locked/media/ch08/08_12ATPCycle.
jpg - Bing.

Figure 44. Metabolic pathways.

In both pathways energy plays an important and crucial role.

But, if we now reconsider, based on the alternative definition of *energy as flows of packages*, what will happen and what will the Transformer look like?

First, today we have this model explaining the pathways of metabolism:

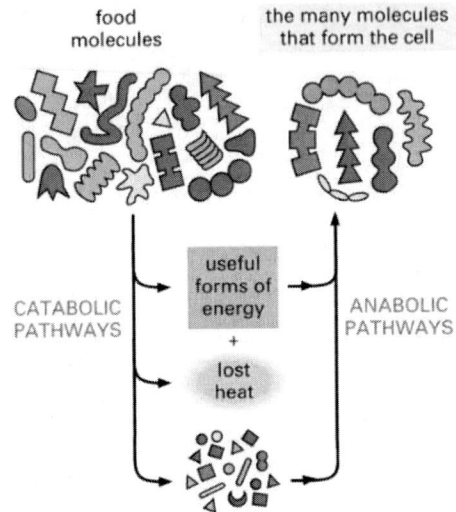

Source: imgurl:https://i.servimg.com/u/f35/17/30/76/23/buildi10.png - Bing.

Figure 45. Processes of metabolism.

The Transformer, in a simplified model, might look like this:

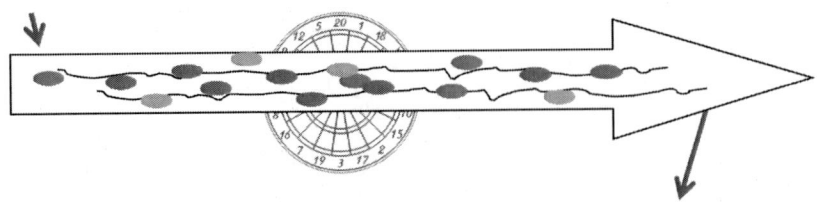

Figure 46. The Transformer.

A transformer replaces ATP synthase and sodium-potassium pump and the concept energy.

Now we must show how molecules transforms via the Transformer and its *mechanism directing and leading the packages*, e.g., protons, electrons and nutrient molecules, within the cells in the human body and also show how new molecules occur.

Let us use this established model:

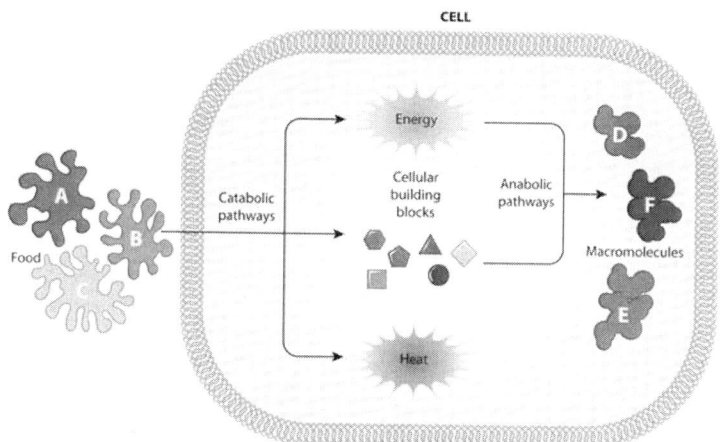

Source: Anabolic & Catabolic Pathways - Principle of Biochemistry (weebly.com).

Figure 47. Contemporary view of catabolic and anabolic reactions.

Now, let's cut out ATP, ADP, P and energy, then we get this pathway:

Complex molecules of glycogen, proteins and triglycerides, change via transformation to simple molecules of glucose, amino acids, glycerol and fatty acids, and change back to complex molecules as well as waste.

Of course we are back to the Transformer and its functionality. (Please remember the huge importance of the Transformer, in all parts of reality, such as gravitation and black holes, as I have investigated in previous books.)

What Is a Transformer?

Now the concept of homeostasis is replaced by the concept *system of flow*. Then we have to show an alternative model, which transforms mass to new molecules.

Let us start with the different parts needed, such as:

1. The shape and its walls
2. Masses in terms of particles and packages
3. How 1 and 2 coincide and consociate.

This solution is also based on the postulate: if the relation is superior, there will be no cause and effect between the parts.

Why, then, are some chemical components coactive and synergetic and why is this not the case with other components?

Which properties make this happen?

Hypothesis dealing with transformation of masses:

1. The pathway has properties which direct and guide packages forward.
2. The packages have properties which direct and guide the packages forward, i.e., catalyst function with help from enzymes.
3. There is interaction between the pathway and the packages, i.e., they are woven together and interconnected.

Then, how can we identify the properties and the interaction to find out which hypothesis is valid?

Which properties have a pathway in order to direct flows of packages?

How is a pathway constructed in order to direct flows of packages to their destinations?

How can a pathway create new cells?

What will it look like when an image is made out of flows, where all flows are connected to each other? For example, how the structure of DNA is related to flows in the cell and how the mitochondria are related to flows from outside. But most important is how the entire system of flows look like throughout the cell.

Since it is hypothesis 2 which is the answer of contemporary science, we focus on hypotheses 1 and 3.

One possible illustration to start with:

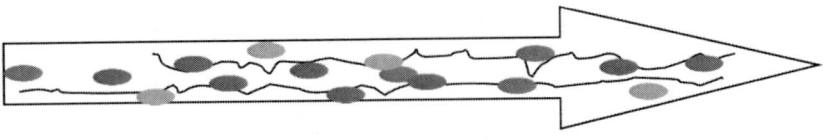

Figure 48. The weave between pathway, infrastructure and packages.

Let us start with an analogy from man-made roads and cars. When cars are driven on any road, they will behave according to road signs. It is not the cars themselves which decide where to go, it is the traffic signs and rules of traffic.

How Mass Moves in the Human Body

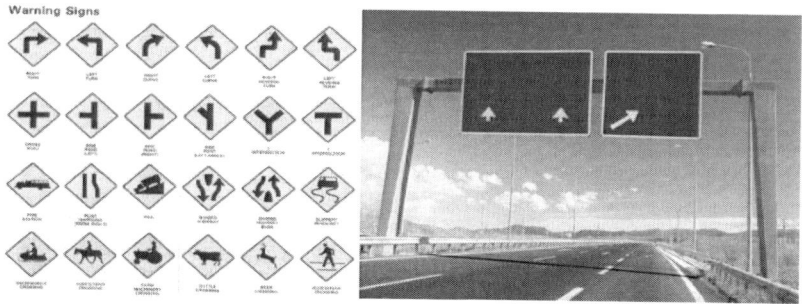

Figure 49. Traffic analogy.

Then imagine that it is the same in the pathways of a cell, e.g., trucks to the left and cars to the right, then separating different masses from each other. Please use images below for your fantasy and imagination …

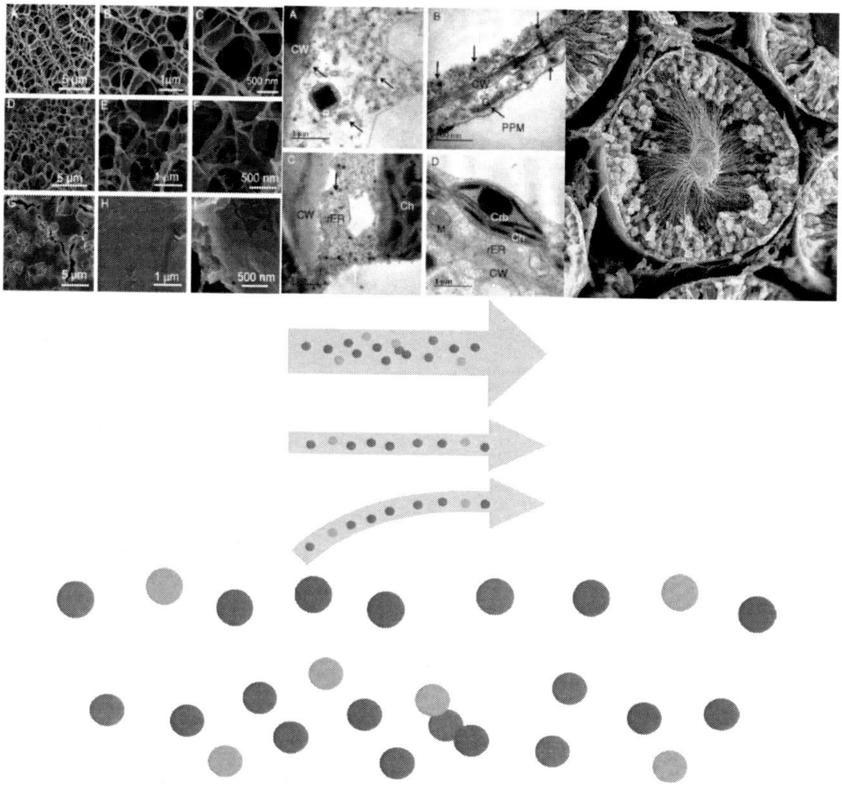

Figure 50. Images of pathways.

Pathways in the cell via electron microscope and inspiring electron microscope pictures.

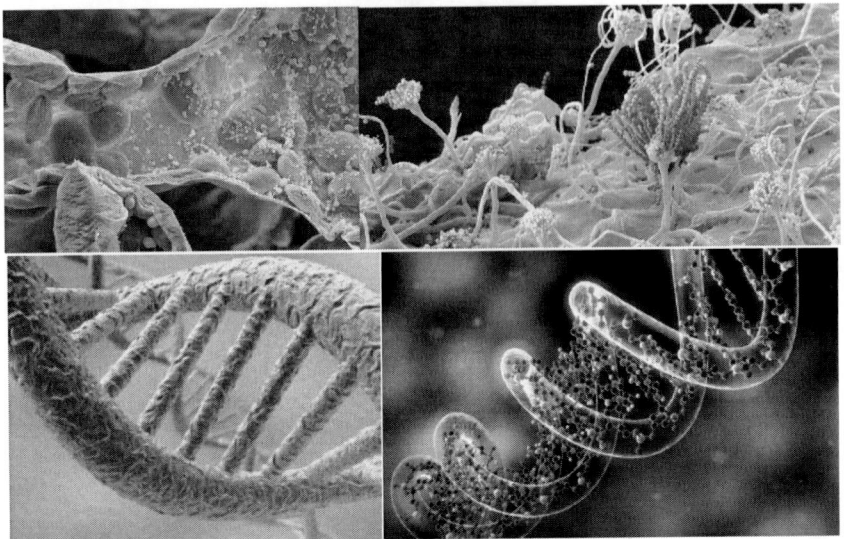

Source: Electron microscope pictures of pathways of DNA – Bildsökresultat (yahoo.com).

Figure 51. Electron microscope pictures of pathways of DNA.

My guess is that hypothesis no. 3 will win.
To be continued ...

Chapter 8

The Principle Applied to ATP Synthase and Sodium-Potassium Pump

We need to find the most efficient and simple pathways within the human body, since that is how nature functions, straight on forward. By using Occam's razor in dealing with scientific concepts, we might find the simplicity of reality.

What manifests as energy is the flow of packages, i.e., R→E, which was demonstrated in Chapter 2.

So, the use of the concept energy is not needed and cannot be used. Why?

First, we have to deal with two requirements or stipulations that must be fulfilled for a theory to be complete:

1. *"Every element of the physical reality must have a counterpart in the physical theory,"* as Albert Einstein proposed.
2. *Every concept has to represent the physical reality directly.*

$E = mc^2$ consists of four concepts, where E, m and c^2 are explicit, while c is implicit, i.e., c is not mentioned directly, only via c^2.

Two important concepts for the theory of relativity are c and c^2, where c is the speed of light and is the fastest anything can travel according to Einstein, i.e., c = 300.000.000 m/s.

Then, c^2 is the speed of light squared, i.e., c^2 = 90.000.000.000.000.000 m/s.

The speed of light is c, which means that c^2 is pure mathematics since it does not have any direct representation in the reality, which is needed due to the requirements or stipulations 1 and 2, i.e., c^2 is not valid.

Then the conclusion is:

1. The equation $E = mc^2$ is not valid. It is only the element *m* of the physical reality that has a counterpart in the physical theory.
2. The equation $E_0 = m_0 c^2$ is not valid.

$E = mc^2$ is Einsteins interpretation of energy, i.e., mass has energy. The speed of light is c, which means that c^2 is pure mathematics since it does not have any direct representation in reality, which is needed due to the stipulation that *every concept has to represent reality directly.* So c^2 is not valid in reality. The same goes for the concept E. Furthermore, in Nature there is no rest energy E_0. In Nature there is no rest mass m_0. The equation $E_0 = m_0 c^2$ is as a consequence not valid. We can also notice that none of the concept's E, m_0 and c^2 fulfils the criterion stipulated by Einstein, namely that "every element of the physical reality must have a counterpart in the physical theory." E is energy in existing theories. Now a, b, c, d ... are units and R is the relation between a, b, c, d ... The consequence is that R will replace E: $E = R$, $E = aRb$, $E = m_1 R m_2$, $E_{1-n} = R_{1-n}(a,b)$; $E_{1-n} = R_{1-n}$; So, based on aRb, we understand that the formula $E = mc^2$ has many difficulties, for this reason: the concept of energy is not a direct representation of reality and is therefore not a valid scientific concept. To use the concept energy as representation seems to be a detour, while the concept of package goes straight to the point, which is in likeness with the stipulation *"every concept has to represent reality directly,"* as made in this book.

A definition of energy as flows of packages changes the view of metabolism, ATP synthase and the sodium-potassium pump, which now is supposed to take energy from the ATP synthase. It is the flows of packages that run cellular processes; this is how food, via the Transformer, is transformed into new molecules, such as proteins, lipids, nuclear acids and carbohydrates.

It is dramatic and it changes our contemporary view of the human body's basic functions.

The new concept Transformer will replace both the ATP synthase and the sodium-potassium pump.

Let us now explore the idea behind the scientific explanation of ATP synthase and give an alternative interpretation based on the principle of relations.

A scientist, like any man, can only observe a small part of reality, even by using a microscope or a telescope. Beyond a certain size of nanometre or of lightyears our apparatus and senses cannot help us to see *how reality behaves.*

Even though science has shown that phenomena such as the ATP synthase and sodium-potassium pump are true objects, existing in reality, and science has shown how they behave, no one has ever seen them directly. They are indeed known by indirect proofs and equations, and this can be the phenomenon of Plato's cave. Furthermore, indirect proofs cannot handle the behaviour of reality; they are at best fixed images. The most famous image of ATP synthase[13]:

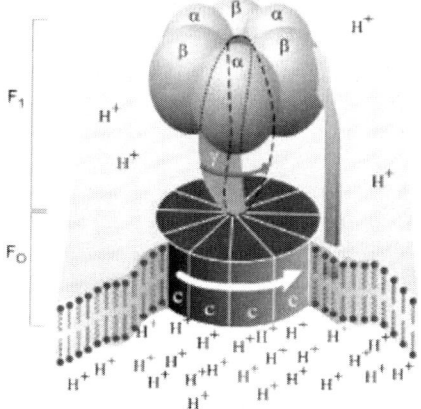

Figure 52. ATP.

One often used image of the sodium-potassium pump:

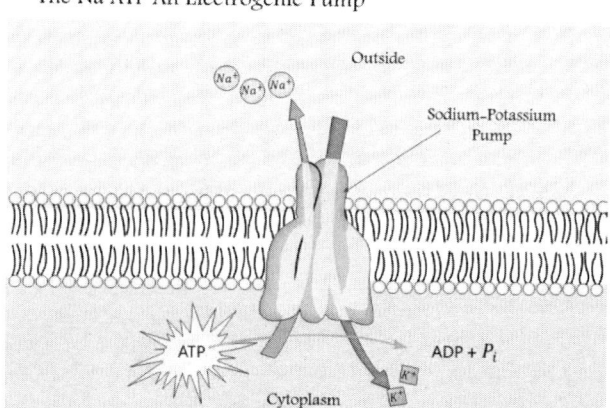

Source: imgurl:https://www.slideteam.net/media/catalog/product/cache/1280x720/ 0/9/0914_the_na_k_atpase_an_electrogenic_pump_medical_images_for_power point_Slide01.jpg - Bing.

Figure 53. Sodium-potassium pump.

---

[13] Synthase. https://www.nobelprize.org/prizes/chemistry/1997/9171-pressmeddelande-nobel priset-i-kemi-1997/.

Then, combining the two, it looks very complicated, as the image below shows:

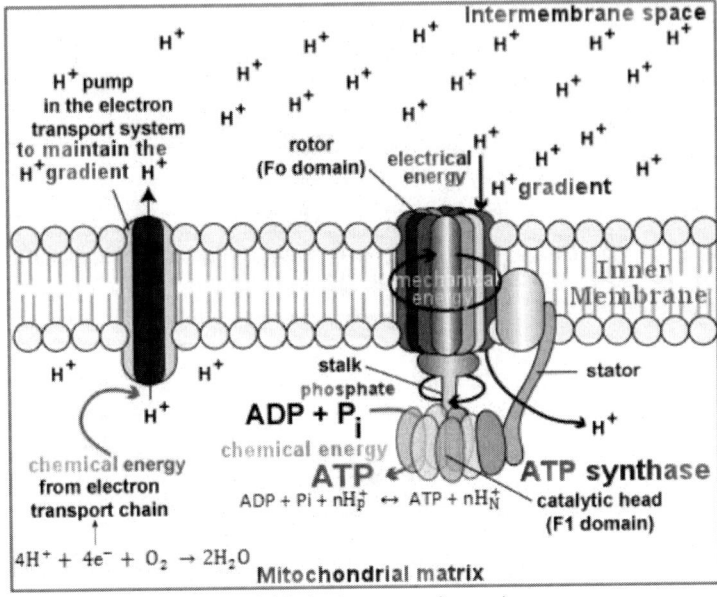

Source: I10-75-ATP.png (451×362) (universe-review.ca).

Figure 54. ATP synthase and sodium-potassium pump working.

At this stage, remember that Nature cannot behave without simplicity and efficiency. Every answer to the mysteries of the Universe, Nature and of the Human body MUST be based on simplicity and beauty. So far, this is not the case when it comes to the ATP synthase and the sodium-potassium pump.

Are they based on optical illusions and invalid equations?

The short answer is YES.

Then the relation between ATP Synthase and the sodium-potassium pump is supposed to be that the sodium-potassium pump uses energy from ATP to pump Na+ out of the cell and K+ into the cell: this is not valid.

At this stage we notice the use of the concept *energy*, which is not valid, and the use of the concept *reverse*, which is not valid.

The questions I want to raise are these:

1. *Does ATP synthase actually exist?*
2. *Does the sodium-potassium pump really exist?*

The Principle Applied to ATP Synthase and Sodium-Potassium Pump

But before answering these questions, we will have to study how ATP synthase is explained and its effects on the sodium-potassium pump, as told by contemporary science:

The function of ATP synthase is to produce ATP, adenosine triphosphate, which is an organic compound, i.e., ATP contains carbon-hydrogen bonds.

Contemporary science views ATP synthase as a catalysed reaction, shown as below:

$$ADP + P_i + 3H^+_{out} \rightleftharpoons ATP + H_2O + 3H^+_{in}$$

ADP consists of $C_{10}H_{15}N_5O_{10}P_2$ and ATP consists of $C_{10}H_{16}N_5O_{13}P_3$.

The reversible reaction, i.e., $\rightleftharpoons$, means equilibrium, i.e., balance and no net change between the components, as explained by the constant K_{eq}.

K_{eq} is the equilibrium constant expressing the ratio of products and reactants at equilibrium.

The meaning is that if a system is not at equilibrium, the system itself will direct moves towards equilibrium.

However, I wish to challenge this notion.

In the case of ATP synthase, these equations and their images reflect each other, i.e., the image is a mirror of the formula. Is it possible that these mirrors are illusions and that we only see what our minds are programmed to see?

An Alternative Interpretation

Based on the Principle of Relations, the logic of ATP synthase is not valid, since the concepts "conjunction," "disjunction," "negation" and "implication," in combination with truth function and the statements of fixed atomic facts and elementary propositions, tell us that there are no values which are true or false, except at a certain point of time. Then the reversible reaction, $\rightleftharpoons$, is not valid and equilibrium does not exist.

Then, when we apply the logic of aRb to our understanding of ATP synthase, the conclusion is different:

1. There are flows of packages in one direction only, e.g., flows of packages are transported into our cells.
2. Equilibrium does not exist in nature.

3. The symbol ⇌ and its meaning of "reversible" reaction is not valid.
4. Carbon-hydrogen bonds do not exist, since it is flows of packages that fulfil the task.

Flows of packages through the body are enabled by the blood pressure securing continuous flows throughout the body.

The circulatory system manages the flow of packages, consisting of blood with its contents of nutrients, such as amino acids and oxygen, waste and carbon-dioxide, which are all transported by vessels.

As it seems, *the blood-pressure resulting from the heart pumping is enough* to fulfil the function of supplying the cells and mitochondria with what is needed and then to clean up and transport the waste. This happens in a continuous performance.

Then, is the ATP synthase, the so-called molecular machine, an illusion? Where can we see this "Nano machine"? Are there any photos of this phenomenon? Is it only an image made by man? As it seems, it is only an image made by man.

Based on the principle of relations both the image and the equations are illusions.

To further understand how the theory of relations impacts the ATP synthase we must find out all connections in the body and how all flows depend on each other.

Based on $X = aRb$ and $S = ap_{1-n}b$, any system is and can be described as complex flows. We might call them wave functions, since a wave function is a flow of masses. It functions as a logistic system. Any (transportation-) system has the same logic. It contains instructions as to how masses are delivered. There are addresses, carriages, details of how the masses are to be loaded and unloaded, sizes of the masses, how the masses fit into different parts of the transport system, calls for masses, "doors" to the cover of a system, and a mechanism to open "doors." At all points of delivery the masses will change appearance. They will look different. They will be transformed.

We call the mechanism of transformation a *Transformer*. The Transformer transforms incoming packages, such as the molecule of carbonic acid CH_2O_3, the molecule of sugar $C_{12}H_{22}O_{11}$, the molecule of protein $C_9H_{11}NO_3$, the molecule of fat $C_{18}H_{34}O_2$ and the molecule of oxygen O_2.

The model below is an overview and conceptualisation of the role the Transformer plays in the human body:

The Principle Applied to ATP Synthase and Sodium-Potassium Pump 69

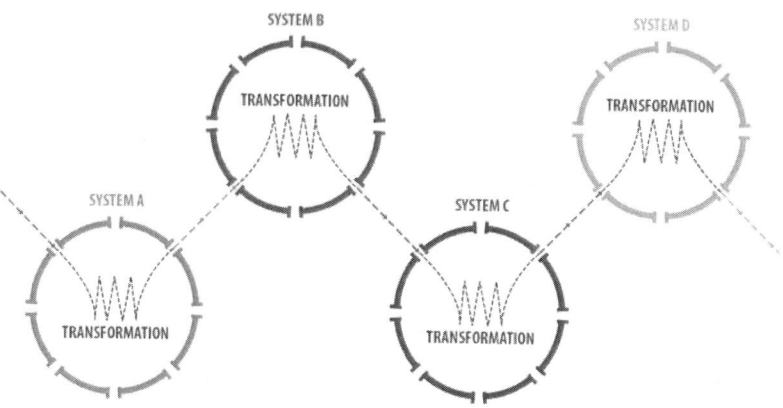

Figure 55. Systems hanging together transforming packages.

The gates are crucial and important, and they can schematically be shown as in this model:

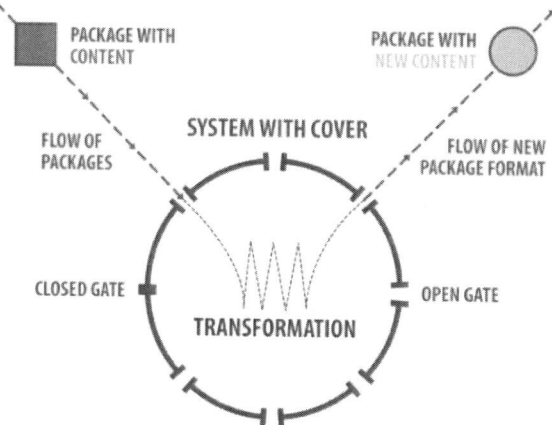

Figure 56. Transformation of packages.

Now, what will the Transformer look like and how will it behave in order to transform packages?

The circulatory system manages the flow of packages, consisting of blood with its contents of nutrients such as amino acids, oxygen, waste and carbon dioxide, which are all transported by vessels, ending in the cell.

The question to be asked now is whether the blood pressure itself is enough to fulfil the function of supplying the "end-stations" in the cell, e.g., mitochondria, and then move out the waste. Or does the cell need the molecular machine?

Based on the principle of relations the hypothesis is that there is only one specific pathway for every piece of mass; i.e., when any particle approaches the membrane of a cell, the structure of the cell will accept the one that fits.

This goes for every membrane, the outer and inner membranes for all cells, as well as for all levels of any system, e.g., the entire human body and any specific organ.

Then, as one consequence, the so-called "Brownian motor," based on the so-called "Brownian motion," does not exist and cannot do so, since randomness is impossible. If randomness, in terms of desultory and casual events, occurs, then the flow of packages will be damaged.

The Brownian Motion

When comparing how the principle of relations finds the answer and how contemporary science finds the answer, there are two quite different theories dealing with the so-called Brownian motion.

The random movement of particles in fluids is called Brownian motion. When particles in a fluid collidewith fast-moving molecules the result is a random motion of these particles. The motion is not deterministic, i.e., the particles have what is called a random walk.

First, I want to quote Einstein: "I, at any rate, am convinced that He (God) does not throw dice." Einstein in 1940 was pessimistic about finding the logical foundation for the theoretical basis of physics and wrote: "Thus it is probably out of the question that any future knowledge can compel physics again to relinquish our present statistical theoretical foundation in favour of a deterministic one which would deal directly with physical reality."

Now, it seems that Einstein embraced both views, i.e., the deterministic view and the random/probability view.

Is it possible to bridge these seemingly opposed views?

To illuminate the concepts of determinism and randomness I present three new postulates:

1. Nothing exists in isolation, i.e., everything exists in relations.
2. Every concept has to represent the physical reality directly.

The Principle Applied to ATP Synthase and Sodium-Potassium Pump

3. The physical reality possesses different levels.

Postulate 3 implies three levels as mentioned in Chapter 1:

1. The fundamental level, which can be difficult to observe.
2. The surface level, which can be seen, by microscope, telescope or with our eyes.
3. The conceptual level, using established scientific concepts, but also new concepts, as used by the Principle of Relations.

Before we solve the problem by using concepts that directly represent the physical reality, we need a different theoretical approach.

Please be prepared for reiteration once more. Based on the first postulate we conclude that all parts and entities in the Universe hang together.

The concept of relation relates to reality by demonstrating that there are relations between all parts in the Universe, formalized as aRb, where:

1. a, b, c ... are any system, subsystem, unit or part, in any field of the Universe, e.g., suns, planets, moons, galaxies, quarks, leptons, hadrons, mesons, baryons, nuclei, atoms and molecules.
2. The relation R is a flow (wave) of packages, p_{1-n}, between a, b, c ... in any field of the Universe.

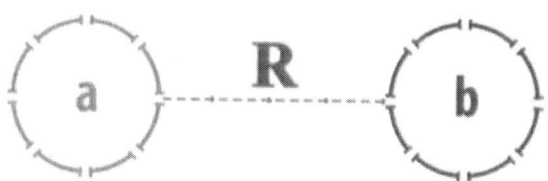

Figure 57. The basic model of relations.

Based on the postulate - *Nothing exists in isolation, i.e., everything exists in relations* - in combination with 1 and 2 above, The Principle of Relations is X = aRb, where X stands for E (Energy), G (Gravitation) and F (Force).

Between all systems and between all parts of any system, S, there is a continuous flow of packages, and the formula is: $S = ap_{1-n}b$.

In experiments using a microscope it is possible to make visible particles with activity, and then verify theories of the Brownian motion, as was done with Einstein's theory.

Einstein used the kinetic theory, KT, to calculate the probability, P, of a particle's movement over a certain distance, x, during some time, t, where the diffusion, D, is known.

Now we have two theories, both aspiring to explain the motion of particles, i.e., the random theories and the theory of relations, where the second is deterministic and the first is based on the postulate of randomness.

How, then, does aRb explain the motion of particles?

At *the fundamental level there are flows of packages*, e.g., rivers or winds that carry the smaller particles from one place to another, i.e., aRb. The validity of the random theories cannot be proven in any experiments, since the circumstances are manipulated according to the theory. Within aRb it is Nature that decides, i.e., at the fundamental level, while at *the surface level chaotic motion is admitted*.

Imagine sliding down a helter-skelter, wobbling from side to side, but still on your way down.

The apparently random motion is not random - all particles move from *a* to *b* - even if it looks chaotic. In nature the particles do not move as in an experiment, from one side to another, wobbling back and forth. In Nature there is always a direction for all particles. The experiment has nothing to do with the behaviour of nature.

The conclusion:

1. The Brownian motion, i.e., why particles move, depends on the flow of packages in nature.
2. The question concerning Brownian motion is not relevant.
3. The Kinetic Theory has to be discussed.

The same principle of flow applies to all systems and all levels and all masses of reality, e.g., the Earth, the Universe, the human body, organs and the cell.

Now we are back to the phenomenon of the Transformer.

The blood transports carbohydrates, proteins and fats, and blood cells contain molecules with the content of C, O, H, N, S and P and of course many others. Schematically it can be illustrated like this:

The Principle Applied to ATP Synthase and Sodium-Potassium Pump 73

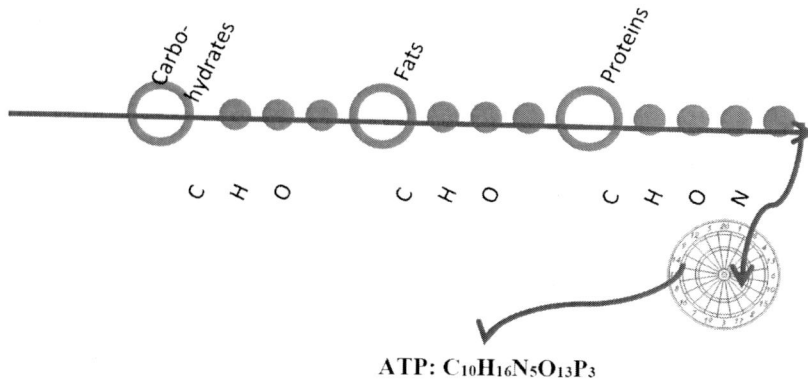

ATP: $C_{10}H_{16}N_5O_{13}P_3$

Figure 58. How new molecules are created via the Transformer.

ATP synthase is a Transformer between molecules using the masses of elementary particles. The conclusion it that ATP synthase does not exist, it is not found in the cell. It is only an imaginary thing, based on wrong and not valid postulates and theories of physics and chemistry.

Chapter 9

The Principle Applied to Inflammation and Its Diseases

In this chapter the principle is applied to the established concepts homeostasis, equilibrium, inflammation and diseases in medicine. The question of how they are related will get a new interpretation.

The introduction of the new principle - *The Principle of Relations* - gives an alternative interpretation of inflammation, homeostasis and diseases.

Based on the basic model below, we can now imagine how flows are being transformed, by the Transformer, in any part of reality.

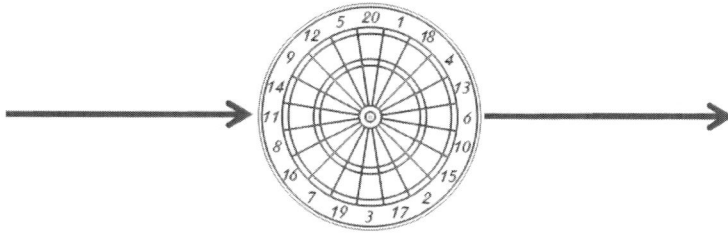

Figure 59. The Transformer.

In this chapter the investigation focuses on the most important concepts involved and how they are related to each other:

1. Inflammation and diseases
2. Homeostasis and its diseases
3. Disruption of homeostasis
4. Flows of packages
5. Gates and their opening or not
6. Transformers

What consequences occur when applying the Principle of Relations and the mechanism of Transformer to inflammation and diseases?

For each system there are gates, i.e., the transformation mechanism by the Transformer, where the content of the packages is transformed for the next level of reality.

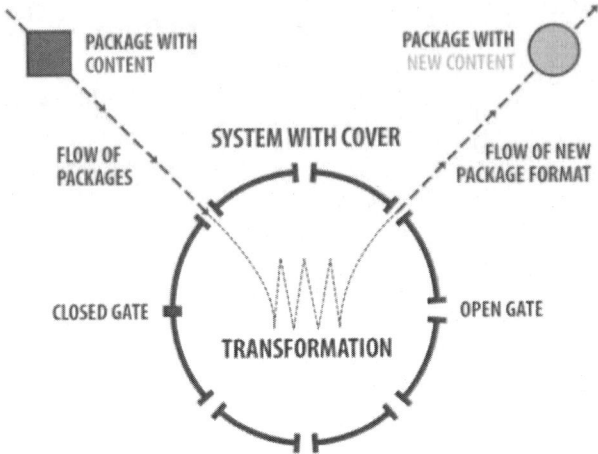

Figure 60. Transformation of packages.

Organs, cells and organelles change and diseases occur when R with its packages arrives or not, via the "doors," i.e., the gates of the cover.

Then behind an inflammation there lies a disordered R. Depending on where the flow-block of R occurs and/or the damaged R occurs, the diseases will be different.

As it seems, chronic inflammation lies behind or at least is connected with diseases such as:

1. Cardiovascular diseases and heart diseases, e.g., AV-block III and heart attack.
2. Metabolic diseases, e.g., diabetes and ALD.
3. Neurodegenerative diseases, e.g., MS, ALS, Dementia, Alzheimer's, Rheumatoid arthritis and Parkinson's.
4. Depression, e.g., Bipolar disorder and suicide.
5. Cancer, e.g., testicular cancer and brain tumour.

The model below gives an overview:

The Principle Applied to Inflammation and Its Diseases

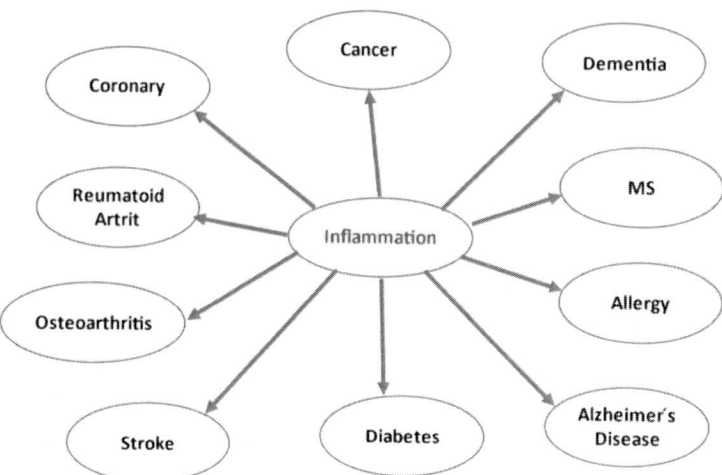

Figure 61. Inflammation's relation towards diseases.

The hypothesis is that the system of flows dominates causing inflammation, while chronic inflammation causes diseases.

First, however, we have to challenge some established concepts, primarily homeostasis, equilibrium and its constant K_{eq}.

Since contemporary science shows that homeostasis and diseases have an inverse relationship, then a disease is related to some imbalance in the human body.

Homeostasis means a body in stability and balance or equilibrium. Sometimes with the addition of dynamic, i.e., dynamic homeostasis and dynamic equilibrium. The net movement must be 0, i.e., what goes in must also go out, the same amount.

Critical is the direction of the movements.

The reversible reaction, i.e., $\rightleftharpoons$, means equilibrium, i.e., balance and no net change between the components, as explained by the constant K_{eq}.

K_{eq} is the equilibrium constant expressing the ratio of products and reactants at equilibrium.

The meaning is that if a system is not at equilibrium, the system itself will direct moves towards equilibrium.

However, I want to challenge this notion.

Equations dealing with ATP synthase in contemporary science views ATP synthase as a catalysed reaction, shown as below:

$$ADP + P_i + 3H^+_{out} \rightleftharpoons ATP + H_2O + 3H^+_{in}$$

ADP consists of $C_{10}H_{15}N_5O_{10}P_2$ and ATP consists of $C_{10}H_{16}N_5O_{13}P_3$.

As we have seen from the Principle of Relations, the concepts flow of packages and transformers, an alternative explanation is possible, i.e., there exists no such thing as homeostasis and equilibrium.

The body is in continuous movement, where each microsecond and at every moment, the systems of the body move, sometimes faster and sometimes slower.

Instead of finding the reason for diseases in lack of homeostasis, we will find damaged flows in and between cells and organs as the reason for diseases.

How, then, concretely, does a flow-block affect the occurrence of an inflammation leading to a disease?

Based on the Principle or Relations, P_R, diseases will occur when R is broken. A broken R is a disorder behind diseases.

The basic questions and statements are:

1. What is the content of R?
2. How is b changed?
3. How is a changed?
4. How does content pass the cover of a and b?
5. When any R, i.e., continuous flow of packages p_{1-n}, is broken, disorder and damage will occur.
6. When any R in S_H is broken, there will be a disease: cancer, high creatinine, AV-blocks, Alzheimer's Disease, kidney failure, stroke, heart attack ...
7. How does gate failure affect R and b, i.e., if the doors between R and b are closed and the interface is out of order?

We know that in normal opening and closing of -ion channels, the flow of ions passes through the membrane of a cell. Our first suspicion is that, for some reason, the gate will not open. When transports in and out of the cell are blocked, the transport of molecules, endocytosis, and waste, exocytosis, cannot be performed.

The Principle Applied to Inflammation and Its Diseases

Flow-Block as a Cause of Diseases

Based on P_R, diseases will occur when R is broken. A broken R is a disorder behind diseases, such as:

- AV-block III
- Stroke
- Heart attack and cardiac infarction
- Alzheimer's disease (AD)
- Schizophrenia
- Kidney failure
- Pain, e.g., in spine, bedpan and muscles
- Cancer.

Flow-Block as a Cause of Alzheimer's Disease (AD)

The model of Alzheimer's disease:

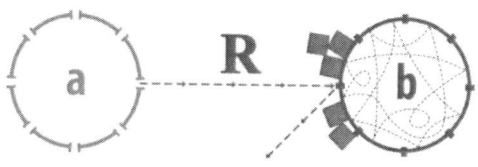

Figure 62. Alzheimer's disease.

So far, the facts, based on science, which correspond to the model of aRb, are:

1. Amyloid, plaques and neurofibrillary tangles are involved.
2. Loss of neurons and synapses.
3. Inflammation.
4. Lower levels of neurotrophic factors and the brain-derived neurotrophic factor, BDNF, (protein).
5. The activity of the neurotransmitter Alpha-7 nicotinic receptor (protein) is modulated by BDNF.

Flow-Block as a Cause of Cancer

When gates are closed, no packages can either come in or leave the cell. Then the cell will be destroyed inside, and outside it the packages will be crowded.

When R is damaged, this will happen, shown by the model over cancer:

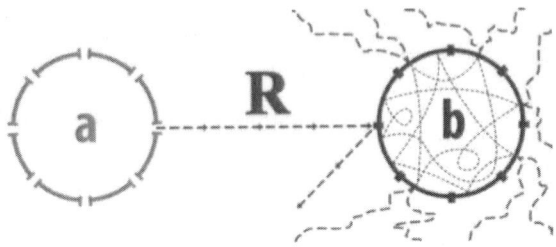

Figure 63. The model of cancer.

The thesis in established science is that damage of DNA causes cancer. However based on P_R it is not genetic disorder that causes and disrupts the cells' normal functioning, since genetic disorder, if there is any, at the first point is caused by a flow-block or damaged R, i.e., damaged flows of packages, in the cell.

So, how can a gate recover from inactivity?

Straight to the Point

Malfunction flows cause inflammation, which causes diseases.

1. How to map, measure and understand the status of flows?
    1.1. CRP
    1.2. Ion-rate
    1.3. Blood pressure
    1.4. ...

2. How to contain all continuous flows in the body?
    2.1. Life style 1-2-3 ...
    2.2. "Drugs" via nano?
    2.3. ...

Now, the difficult search for the answers.

How to Cure Inflammation?

Based on aRb, the flow must function again. It can be done by exercise, hard exercise. Then the blood system will, over time, build new vessels occurring in the bloodstream and take away blocks.

To be continued in Chapter 14 ...

Chapter 10

The Principle Applied to Cancer

In this chapter an alternative explanation of what causes cancer is introduced.

There are two dominating theoretical bases for understanding the mechanisms of cancer:

1. The architecture of the genome is understood as explaining how cancers occur. The hypothesis of contemporary science focuses on genes as the cause of cancer, i.e., a bottom-up approach.
2. The hypothesis in this book introduces damaged flows to be the cause of cancer. The hierarchy of flows means that if a superior system collapses, then all subordinate systems will collapse and cancer can occur, i.e., a top-down approach.

Then, two different approaches dispute. The first starts at the level of a gene and the second starts at the level outside genes, inside the cell organelles or outside the cell, i.e., *asking if cancer starts inside the cell or if cancer starts outside the cell.*

The Principle of Relations claims that DNA is an infrastructure, i.e., *the mechanism which directs and leads packages of molecules,* to be called *transformer,* i.e., DNA transforms masses.

The Principle of Relations claims that the structure of the chemical components A, T, G and C organizes how incoming masses are built. At a certain size, the cell has to divide, since it cannot handle too much incoming masses. Then, *genetic information is the physical structure of the chemical components A, T, G and C.* Even if sequences of A, T, G and C can be considered as a four-letter alphabet, it is concrete, solid and coactive chemical components, which allow flows to move in a specific order, guided by the structure. When cells have to divide due to lack of space, new cells occur guided by the structure.

Based on this conclusion, it is not genes that control either when cells divide or when cells grow: it is the flow of nutrition's. It is not oncogenes that cause cancer, it is malfunctioning metabolism and damaged flows of nutrition's molecules.

The first hypothesis is often used in research, as the following:

"With the vast trove of data about human DNA generated by the Human Genome Project and other genomic research, scientists and clinicians have more powerful tools to study the role that multiple genetic factors acting together and with the environment play in much more complex diseases. These diseases, such as cancer, diabetes, and cardiovascular disease constitute the majority of health problems in the United States. Genome-based research is already enabling medical researchers to develop improved diagnostics, more effective therapeutic strategies, evidence-based approaches for demonstrating clinical efficacy, and better decision-making tools for patients and providers. Ultimately, it appears inevitable that treatments will be tailored to a patient's particular genomic makeup. Thus, the role of genetics in health care is starting to change profoundly and the first examples of the era of genomic medicine are upon us."

The second hypothesis claims that damaged flows cause cancer. The hypothesis starts with a new principle in our understanding of the human body. Please accept one more reiteration, needed in this section for comparing.

The principle is based on three stipulated postulates:

1. Nothing exists in isolation; everything exists in relations.
2. Movement is a property of reality.
3. Every concept has to represent reality directly and concretely.

Based on the postulate - Nothing exists in isolation; everything exists in relations - in combination with 1 and 2 above, the principle is

$X = aRb,$

where X is any system, inflammation and disease.

Between all systems and between all parts of any system, S, within the human body, there are continuous flows of packages p_{1-n}, i.e., $R = p_{1-n}$. The formula will be thus:

$S = ap_{1-n}b$

R contains p_{1-n} and the function of R is: $R = \sum p_{1-n} = p_1 + p_2 + p_3 \ldots p_n$

This content will over time change any structure a, b, c in the human body, from the lowest element in the cells to relations between subsystems. Within the body there is complex R_{1-n}.

Now we might combine pathway and flows, since flows need pathways, but still, some flows are superior, as hypothesis 2 claims based on article 3.7 above at page 13.

Superior aRb dominates affecting subordinate aRb. When any superior aRb is damaged it will affect related aRb. If any superior aRb collapses, any related subordinate aRb will collapse as well. This is the top-down approach.

Based on the Principle or Relations diseases will occur when R is broken. A broken R is a disorder behind diseases.

Consequently cancer and degenerative diseases are not caused by genes, they are caused by damaged superior aRb, i.e., damaged flows.

Flow-Block as a Cause of Cancer

When gates are closed, no packages can either come in or leave the cell. Then the cell will be destroyed inside, and outside it the packages will be crowded.

The basic logic is this model:

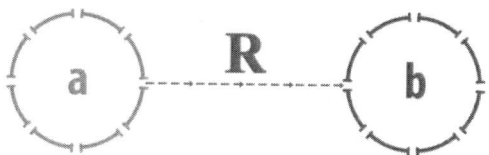

Figure 64. The basic model of relations.

When R is damaged, this will happen, shown by the model over cancer:

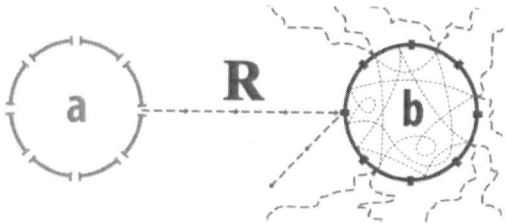

Figure 65. The model of cancer.

The thesis in established science is that damage of DNA causes cancer. However based on the Principle of Relations it is not genetic disorder that causes and disrupts the cells' normal functioning, since genetic disorder, if there is any, at the first point is caused by a flow-block or damaged R, i.e., damaged flows of packages, in the cell.

This investigation focuses on finding the lowest common denominator causing cancer.

Based on the principle of relations' formula X = aRb, we can systematically investigate different types of cancer, following the basic cause; *When any network of tubules is damaged, it will cause cancer:*

1. X = Breast cancer. When the network of blood supply is damaged, it can cause cancer. The systems of arteries and veins have to be investigated to find out where damage can occur.
2. X = Lung cancer. When the network of tubules is damaged, lung cancer will occur. Smoking, radon and asbestos are the most common external environmental circumstances, which then damage the network. It is mostly the tar that cuts off the pathways for the flows.
3. X = Prostate cancer. When the network of connective tissues between glandular tissues is damaged, it may cause cancer. Any system in the human body has to function and normal sex life reduces the risk, based on the theory of aRb; also high risk occurs when this system in not used. The same goes for testicular cancer.
4. X = Kidney cancer. When any network is damaged, cancer can occur.
5. X = Brain cancer. When networks of arteries are damaged, cancer can occur. Since the brain is very complex consisting of many networks, we will start with the so-called Willis Circe, in order to find out how damaged flows of oxygen and nutrition can affect cells.
6. X = Leukaemia. When the infrastructure of bone marrow is damaged, it can cause leukaemia.
7. X = Liver cancer. Since the networks of liver perform complex functions, such as digestion and detoxification, the causes of cancer are numerous. At this stage it is too early to identify all possible causes from networks, since many forms of liver cancer have spread to the liver from other areas of the body. However, we need to mention the lobules of the liver, i.e., the portal triad and its connective tissue, when damaged flow can cause cancer.

8. X = Testicular cancer. Efferent ducts connect the rete testis and its network of tubules carrying sperm from the seminiferous tubules. Anastomoses connect different parts in the testicle when it is normal. If the network becomes damaged, i.e., blocked,cancer will occur.
9. X = Malignant Melanoma. The network which the skin is part of can cause skin cancer. We need to identify how this can happen, e.g., when ultraviolet radiation affects the cells of the skin.
10. X = Pancreatic cancer. We need to identify which are the networks that can be damaged, since there are some; but we might start with anastomoses that join the anterior and posterior branches of the superior pancreaticoduodenal artery.
11. Etc.

As it seems and based on the Principle of Relations, when any flow or network is damaged by obstacles and blocks, the damage will affect cells and cause cancer.

Why, where and how do damaged flows and networks occur?

1. Gate failure of cell.
2. Microtubule damage.
3. Damaged flow contents.
4. Damaged anastomosis cannot fulfil its function and flows will stop. In all parts of the human body anastomosis is present, e.g., the Willis Circle, within testicles and in the inferior epigastric artery and the superior epigastric artery.
5. Combination of 1-4.

By looking through the lens of this principle, we are mostly looking at the R_{1-n}, i.e., at networks of relations consisting of flows and their contents.

First, we focus on the concept and content of the cytoskeleton, consisting of microtubules, microfilaments and intermediate filaments. The functions of the cytoskeleton are complex but, dealing with diseases of cancer, we focus on the dynamic network, i.e., the uptake of extracellular material (endocytosis), and organizing organelles. The cytoskeleton consists of filaments and microtubules, as the image below shows:

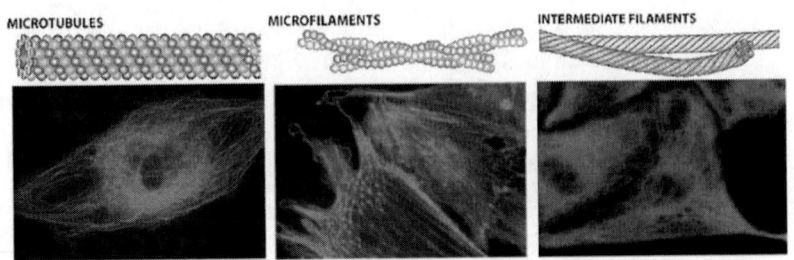

Source: Network of cytoskeletal filaments [5,8] .... | Download Scientific Diagram (researchgate.net).

Figure 66. Networks of the cell.

The Logistic System and Its Flows within the Cell

The most important parts and concepts are the following:

1. Cytoskeleton
2. Microtubules
3. Microfilaments
4. Intermediate filaments
5. Axonal transport
6. Integrin

We know that, in normal opening and closing of ion channels, the flow of ions passes through the membrane of a cell. Our first suspicion is that the gate will not open, for some reason. So, how can a gate recover from inactivity?

We will now focus on how damaged gates will affect the cytoskeletons' contact with the membrane and extracellular material.

How, then, to connect the cytoskeleton to extracellular material?

The receptor which connects cytoskeleton to extracellular material is called *integrin*, which looks like a cyclical liaison. Integrins are receptors at the surface of the cell, fulfilling its mediation.

The image below shows how this is made, where E=extracellular space; I=intracellular space; P=plasma membrane, i.e., the function of transmembrane receptor:

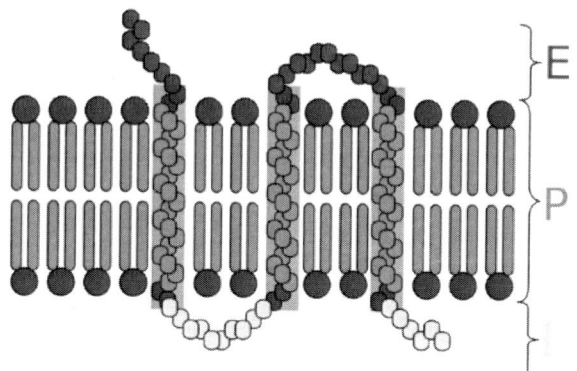

Source: Cell surface receptor - Wikipedia.

Figure 67. Integrin.

Integrin connects the cytoskeleton and the extracellular matrix. Based on aRb, damaged flows create cancer and if the integrin does not function it can be one possible cause for cancer. Then, the figure below can guide us to the first possible cause:

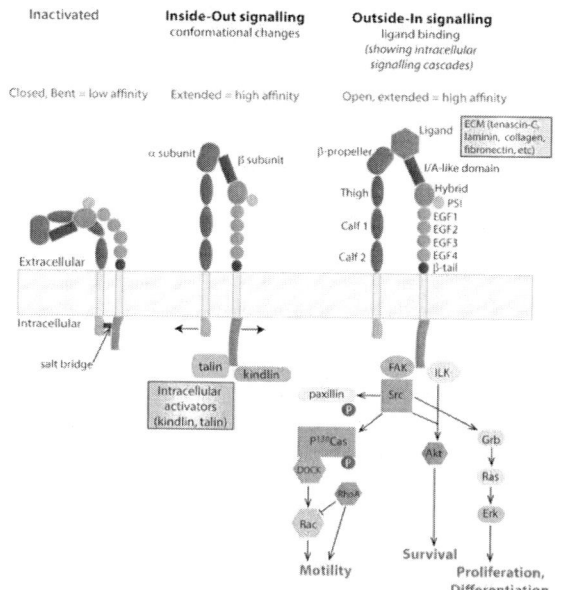

Source: Cells | Free Full-Text | Integrin Activation: Implications for Axon Regeneration | HTML (mdpi.com).

Figure 68. Integrin's network.

The figure describes the integrin Structure and Activation. "Activation of integrin heterodimers leads to intracellular signalling cascades and resulting processes such as cell motility, cell survival, cell differentiation, and neurite outgrowth. Schematic representing integrin conformations at the membrane including changes that occur with 'Inside–Out signalling' and 'Outside–In signalling'. An inactivated integrin heterodimer exists with a closed and bent conformation (extracellularly) stabilised by a cytoplasmic salt bridge. This conformation has a very low ligand binding affinity. With Inside–Out signalling, intracellular activators (such as kindlin and talin) bind the β subunit cytoplasmic ally and interact/destabilise the salt bridge, leading to an open and extended (active) conformation with increased ligand binding affinity. With Outside–In signalling, binding of a ligand (ECM molecules such as laminin, fibronectin, or tenascin) occurs extracellularly as a result of integrin activation leading to a conformational change to an open and extended (active) conformation with high ligand binding affinity. Individual names of the extracellular domain components have been shown in the Outside–In signalling example for simplicity, with further explanation in the main text." (Source: Cells | Free Full-Text | Integrin Activation: Implications for Axon Regeneration | HTML (mdpi.com))

In the article *Integrin Activation: Implications for Axon Regeneration*, the authors Menghon Cheah and Melissa R. Andrews also conclude that "As integrins are essential for the proper functioning of a normal and healthy nervous system, translational researchers in the field of axon regeneration have been trying to harvest the use of integrins following a central nervous system (CNS) injury, such as spinal cord injury, in order to recapitulate a developmental growth state that could enhance regenerative growth."

But, how can we find out the function of an integrin, when it is large, complex and linked to many sugar trees? (Integrin - Wikipedia)

Even after many years of research and hundreds of papers, it is not possible to find the structure of integrins.

One attempt is made based on this model, made by Richard O. Hynes. (PII: S0092-8674(02)00971-6 (cell.com).

We are told that "integrins are αβ heterodimes; each subunit crosses the membrane once, with most of each polypeptide (>1600 amino acids in total) in the extracellular space and two short cytoplasmic domains (20-50 amino acids). …"

Then, is the damaged integrin answer to questions about the cause of cancer? And then, how can reparation of integrins prevent and cure cancer?

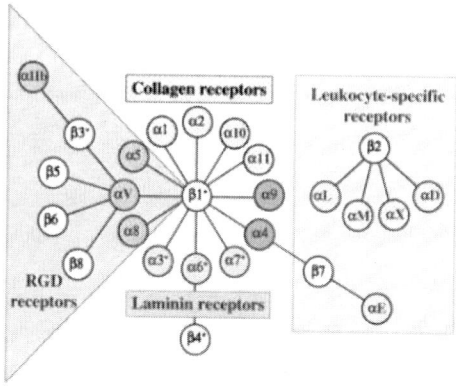

Figure 69. Structure of integrin.

It is obvious that some transformation will fulfil the function of transportation of molecules, but it is not certain that integrin has the answer. So, we might as well, based on the principle of relations, create an alternative solution; as told before, the name is *transformer*. The shape of a transformer, looking like a paddle wheel, will differ depending on where it is located. The image below might stimulate our imagination (the size will be measured in nanometres, approximately 50-200 nm); each number on the wheel can accept only one specific particle from a molecule, e.g., H, N, P, C and O, at the left side, and then a new molecule will occur, e.g., $C_{10}H_{16}N_5O_{13}P_3$, at the right side:

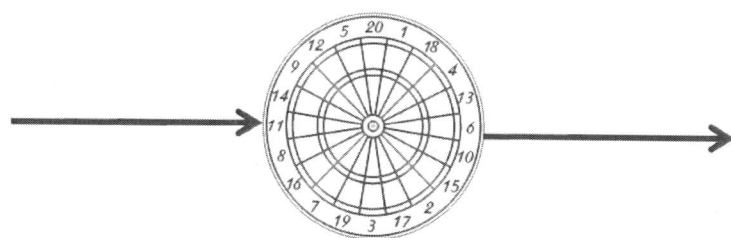

Figure 70. The Transformer.

(It is notable that besides dealing with the human body, throughout reality a transformer functions using the same principal mechanism, e.g., the Earth, the Sun, the Moon, galaxies, black holes, organs and cells in the Human Body).

Outside the cell packages will be crowded and inside the cell chaos will occur, since without any flow of nutrition panic will occur. Then, inside the cell, organelles will reorganize in order to attack its neighbours to find nutrition.

The cancer cell, called malignant tumour, to the right, spreads aggressively invading the surrounding tissues; the cell called benign tumour, at the left, remains self-contained from neighbouring tissue:

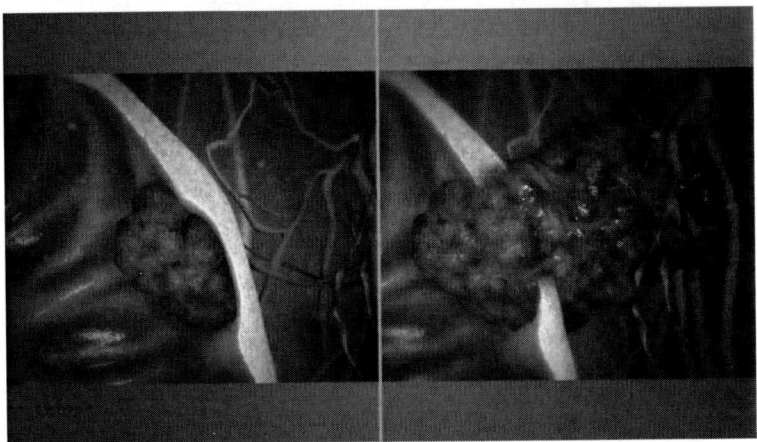

Figure 71. Malignant tumour.

File:Types of tumor cells.jpg - Wikimedia Commons

The size, shape, protein composition, texture and content of the cancer cell is changed.

How, exactly, is the cell reorganized?

The answer is of utmost importance, since then we can find the cause of the change.

Can Mitochondria Cause Cancer?

How do cells grow? Is growth caused by internal structure or is it caused by external structures? Can a cell grow by itself, or does it need extracellular support? What does the combination look like? What role does the nucleus and its DNA in the cell play and what role might the mitochondria play?

The dominant cause of cancer is damaged DNA, according to contemporary science, as we have seen.

Based on X = aRb, damaged flow can create cancer.

How, then, can we find the mechanism behind the behaviour of aggressive cells? Which part in the cell will take control when survival of the cell, caused by damaged flow, is needed?

When a human, a society or a cell is threatened and death might happen, the entire focus will be on survival. So, then, which part in the cell takes this role?

How will mitochondria act if survival of the cell is threatened?

Can the function of mitochondria be used to develop cancer? What is its role in cancer?

Normally the mitochondria fulfil tasks such as producing energy from food and protecting DNA, then securing survival for the cell. Mitochondria is also signalling between cells and cell death.

Let us call the following two hypotheses' numbers 1 and 2:

Hypothesis 1. Let us start with the hypothesis that it is mitochondria that act, and then expand a plan for survival by finding energy by transforming food.

In last decade, research has studied how mitochondrial dysfunction causes many diseases, such as Alzheimer's, diabetes and cancer.

Some support from science, as it seems, for the hypothesis.

Now we have to understand how mitochondria will reorganize in order to get food for energy. What does the action plan look like? What is the content?

Besides hypothesis 1, we can formulate hypothesis 2, dealing with the entire cell.

Hypothesis 2: The entire cell reorganizes in order to get food. What does the action plan look like? What is the content?

Now, let us deal with a possible drug to cure cancer, called a manifold drug.

How, Then, Can We Create a Manifold Drug and Treatment for Cancer?

Starting with molecules and their atoms, we then create a new molecule as a drug for cancer.

The atoms and the molecules are the following:

1. Glutamic acid using the atoms C, H, N, O and its formula $C_5H_9NO_4$
2. Ligands using the atoms H, C, O, o and its formula $HCo(CO)_4$
3. Lysine uses the atoms N, H and its formula $-NH_3^+$
4. The salt bridge uses the atoms H, O, N, R and its formula and function can be seen in these two figures, connecting two halves of the molecular capsule:

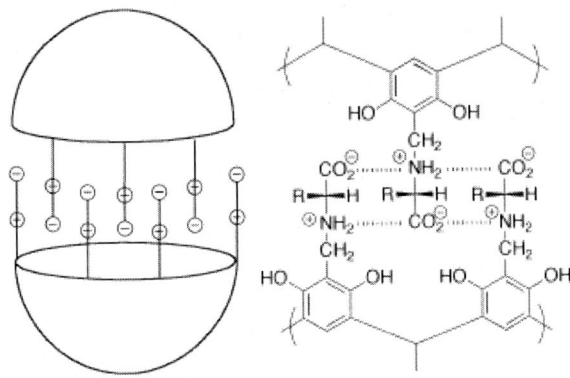

Figure 72. Chemicals of molecular capsule.

It seems obvious that we do not have a full understanding of how mass moves in the human body. Then we have two choices for dealing with drugs and treatment for cancer:

1. By a combination of atoms and molecules, based on what has been told above, create the drug.
2. Accept one superior aRb and by its activation repair the cell.

We have to find the dominant and superior aRb, which dictates the process. We must implement a system for fulfilling flows of atoms and molecules. The flow of C – H – N – O – H – C - O – N – H – H must be restored.

Now we have to find out how to organize this chain C – H – N – O – H – C - O – N – H – H.

Then we have to produce the molecule and find out how to inject it into the human body, i.e., how to put it into the brain.

Of course a huge amount of work has to be done, searching all around the entire human body and all its systems of relations, flows and networks.

Now, I do really hope for help from the scientific society viewing the human body with these new glasses, in the words of Thomas S. Kuhns:

> "...when paradigms change, the world itself changes with them. Led by a new paradigm, scientists adopt new instruments and look in new places. Even more important, during revolutions scientists see new and different things when looking with familiar instruments in places they have looked before." "Nevertheless, paradigm changes do cause scientists to see the world of their research-engagement differently."[14] This is a demanding iterative process engaging hundreds of scientists and thousands of lab tests and clinical trials before the molecule becomes a drug seen as a masterpiece.

---

[14] Thomas S. Kuhn: *The Structure of Scientific Revolutions*. 2012.

Chapter 11

The Principle Applied to Testicular Cancer

In this chapter cancer of testicles will be investigated, based on the Principle of Relations, i.e., how damaged flows cause cancer.

The cause of testicle cancer is unknown. However, most researchers say that cancer is a genetic disease, i.e., changes in genes cause cells to grow abnormally. When cell growth gets out of control, cancer occurs. Many mutations must happen, and in a special order, to develop cancer. How this happens is not known.

In the meantime, we can look at quite different hypotheses, one of which will be presented in this chapter.

First, let us look at one normal testicle, and one testicle with tumour:

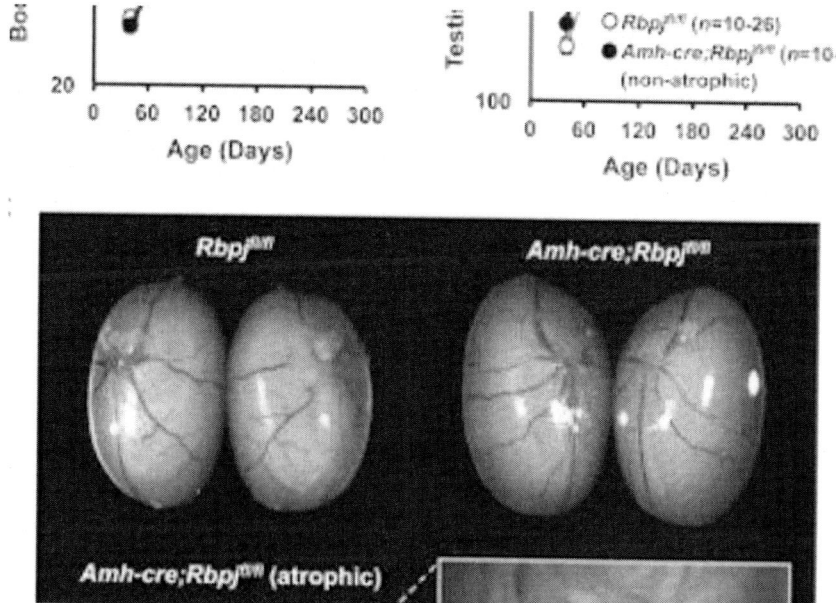

Figure 73. Normal testicles.

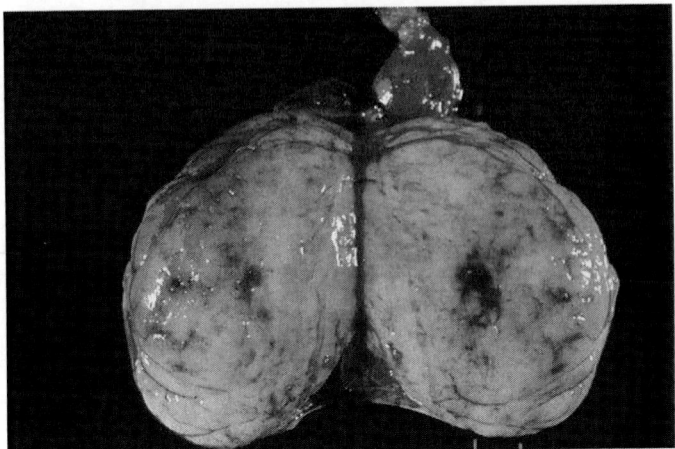

Source: Testicular Cancer Photograph by Cnri/science Photo Library | Fine Art America.

Figure 74. Tumour testicle.

The difference is obvious.
But why and how did cancer occur in the testicle?
Contemporary science has no answer. The cause of cancer is unknown.
We know that cells start to grow with no control and develop abnormalities.
Then, after some time, you will notice that the testicle is bigger and harder. (I had this myself, a surgical amputation was done, followed by radiation. Yes, I did survive, but still very interested – *what really happened?*)

1. The hypothesis of contemporary science focuses on genes to be the cause of cancer, i.e., a bottom-up approach.
2. The hypothesis in this chapter introduces damaged flows to be the cause of cancer, i.e., a top-down approach.

Then, the two different approaches are in conflict. The first starts at the level of a gene and the second starts at the level outside genes, inside the cell organelles or outside the cell, i.e., *asking if cancer starts inside the cell or if cancer starts outside the cell.*
The structure of the chemical components A, T, G and C organizes how incoming masses are built. At a certain size, the cell has to divide, since it cannot handle too many incoming masses. Then, *genetic information is the physical structure of the chemical components A, T, G and C.* Even if

sequences of A, T, G and C can be considered as a four-letter alphabet, they are concrete, solid and coactive chemical components, which allow flows to move in a specific order, guided by the structure. When cells have to divide due to lack of space, new cells occur guided by the structure.

Based on this conclusion, it is not genes that control when cells divide or when cells grow: it is the flow of nutrition. It is not oncogenes that cause cancer, it is malfunctioning metabolism.

How, then, does damaged metabolism cause cancer?

Since we know the answer from the first hypothesis, we do not go any further with it at this point.

The answer from the second hypothesis, in short, goes like this:

When any network of tubules is damaged, it will cause cancer. Efferent ducts connect the rete testis and its network of tubules carrying sperm from the seminiferous tubules. Anastomosis connect different parts in the testicle when it is normal. If the network becomes damaged, i.e., blocked, testicular cancer will occur.

The longer answer goes like this:

It all starts with a new principle for understanding the human body and it is called the Principle of Relations.

Based on the principle X = aRb, we find:

1. X = Cancer. When any network of tubules is damaged, it will cause cancer.
2. X = Testicle cancer. Efferent ducts connect the rete testis and its network of tubules carrying sperm from the seminiferous tubules. Anastomoses connects different parts in the testicle when it is normal. If the network becomes damaged, i.e., blocked, cancer will occur.

Now we have reached the moment of truth.

The Principle of Relations claims that damaged flow dominates causing inflammation, while chronic inflammation causes disease. If damaged flows continue not being repaired, disease will be chronic, i.e., *when any flow is broken or damaged, there will be disorders and diseases, e.g., cancer, AV-block III, Stroke, Alzheimer's and cardiac infarction*[4].

Then, the basic hypothesis for testicular cancer will be: *When any network of tubules is damaged in the testicle, it will cause testicular cancer.*

Now we have to identify all flows in the testicle, using this model (File:Illu testis schematic.jpg - Wikimedia Commons):

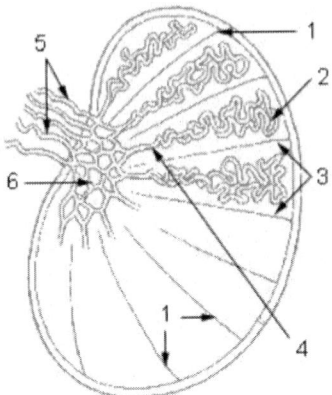

Figure 75. Flows of the testicle.

(1) are the testicular septa; (2) is the convoluted seminiferous tubules; (3) is the testicular lobules; (4) is the straight seminiferous tubules; (5) is the efferent ducts; (6) is the rete testis. Septa (wall) divides tubules

1. The testis septa, its walls, contain lobules of the testicle.
2. The convoluted seminiferous tubules process the producing of sperms.
3. Testicle lobules consist of 300-400 lobules and have conical shape, extending between the mediastinum testis and the tunic seminiferous.
4. The straight seminiferous tubules connect to the rete testis, i.e., anastomosis.
5. The efferent ducts connect the rete testis and its network of tubules carrying sperm from the seminiferous tubules.
6. The rete testis is an anastomosis, connecting different parts in the testicle and reabsorbing fluids.

Now we can expand the hypothesis and make it more detailed: Efferent ducts connect the rete testis and its network of tubules, carrying sperm from the seminiferous tubules, and anastomosis connects different parts of the testicle when it is normal. When the network becomes damaged, i.e., blocked, testicular cancer will occur.

Besides all flows in tubules and the anastomosis, there are flows which go in and out of testicles, such as blood vessels and lymphatic drainage.

Where, is the question, can flow in the testicle be damaged?

What causes the damage?

Then, the basic hypothesis for testicular cancer will be: *When any network of tubules is damaged in the testicle, it will cause testicular cancer.*

Besides all flows in tubules and the anastomosis, there are flows which go in and out of testicles, such as blood vessels and lymphatic drainage.

Wherever any flow is damaged and for whatever reason, disease occurs.

When it comes to testicle cancer, there can be damaged flow caused by drained tubules. If any tubule is not used, it can die or be injured and malfunction, when the case will be living in celibacy. If any blockage occurs, the flow cannot find its destination.

Where, is the question, can flow in the testicle be damaged?

What causes the damage?

Is the damage a blocked tubule or a blocked blood vessel or a duct obstruction?

Now we have to investigate all parts of the testicle. The following images give a start as to where to look:

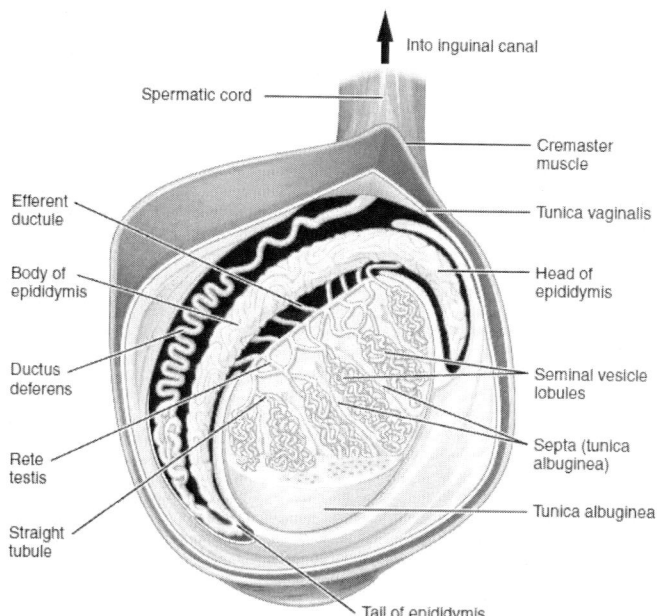

Source: imgurl:https://upload.wikimedia.org/wikipedia/commons/5/55/Figure_28_01_03.JPG - Bing.

Figure 76. Image of a testicle.

The rete testis as shown in micrograph:

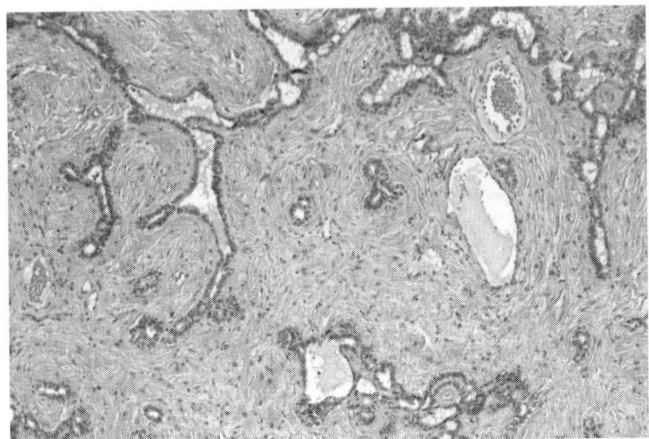

Source: Micrograph of testicle picture – Bildsökresultat (yahoo.com).

Figure 77. Micrograph of testicle.

The seminiferous tubule (right) with sperm (black, tiny, ovoid). H&E stain.

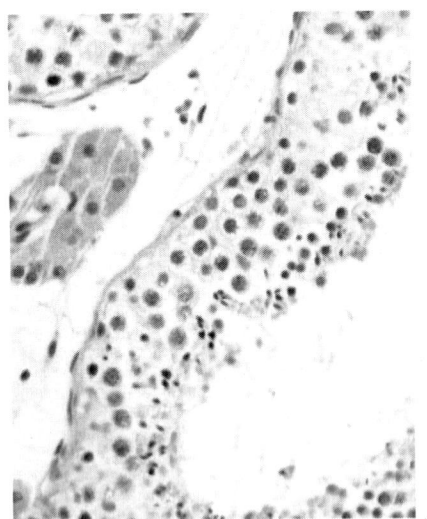

Source: Seminiferous tubule of testicle – Bildsökresultat (yahoo.com).

Figure 78. Seminiferous tubule of testicle.

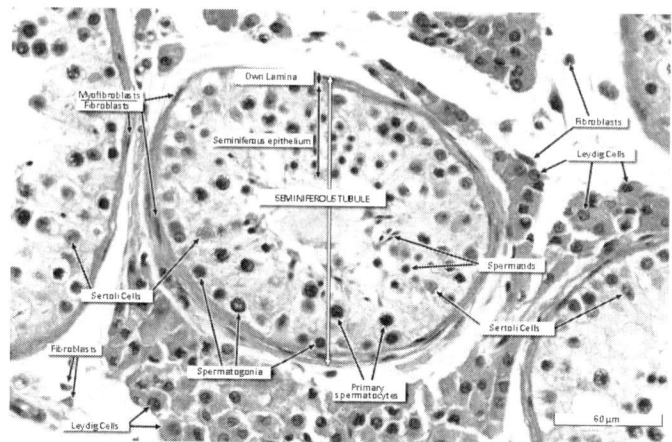

Source: networks of testicle – Bildsökresultat (yahoo.com).

Figure 79. Networks of testicle.

Where in these tubules can obstacles occur and damage flow?
When any flow is damaged by obstacles and blocks, it will affect cells. How?

Outside the cell, packages will be crowded, and inside the cell chaos will occur, since without any flow of nutrition panic will occur. Then, inside the cell, organelles will reorganize in order to attack its neighbours to find nutrition.

The cancer cell, called malignant tumour, to the right, spreads aggressively invading the surrounding tissues; at the left is a benign tumour, which remains self-contained from neighbouring tissue. (File:Types of tumor cells.jpg - Wikimedia Commons):

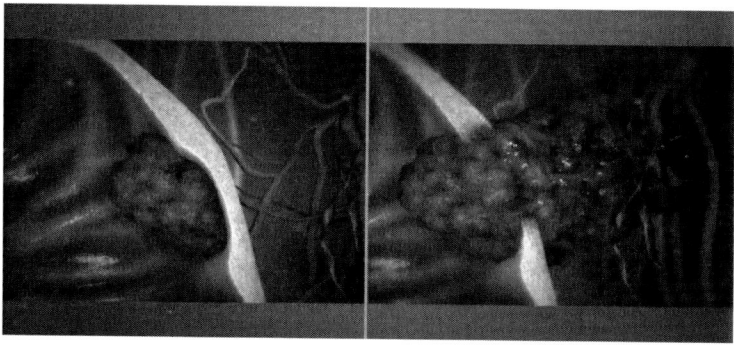

Figure 80. Aggressive tumour.

The size, shape, protein composition, texture and content of the cancer cell is changed.

How, exactly, is the cell reorganized?

The answer is of utmost importance, since then we can find the cause of the change.

Can Mitochondria Cause Cancer?

How do cells grow? Is growth caused by internal structure or is it caused by external structures? Can a cell, by itself, grow or does the cell need extracellular support? What does the combination look like? What role does the nucleus and its DNA play in the cell, and what role might the mitochondria play?

The dominant cause of cancer is damaged DNA, according to contemporary science.

Based on $X = aRb$, damaged flow can create cancer.

How, then, can we find the mechanism behind the behaviour of aggressive cells? Which part in the cell will take control when survival of the cell, caused by damaged flow, is needed?

When a human being, a society or a cell is threatened and death might happen, the entire focus will be on survival. So, then, which part in the cell takes on this role?

How will mitochondria act if survival of the cell is threatened?

Can the function of mitochondria be used to develop cancer? What is its role in cancer?

Usually the mitochondria fulfil tasks such as producing energy from food and protecting DNA, then securing survival for the cell. Mitochondria are also signalling between cells and cell death.

Hypothesis 1. Let us start with the hypothesis that it is mitochondria that act, and then expand a plan for survival by finding energy by transforming food.

In last decade, research has studied how mitochondrial dysfunction causes many diseases, such as Alzheimer's disease, diabetes and cancer.

Some support from science, as it seems, for the hypothesis.

Now we have to understand how mitochondria will reorganize in order to get food for energy. What does the action plan look like? What is the content?

Besides hypothesis 1, we can formulate hypothesis 2, dealing with the entire cell.

Hypothesis 2: The entire cell reorganizes in order to get food. What does the action plan look like? What is the content?

Now, I do really hope for help from the scientific society viewing the human body with these new glasses; in the words of Thomas S. Kuhns:

"...when paradigms change, the world itself changes with them. Led by a new paradigm, scientists adopt new instruments and look in new places. Even more important, during revolutions scientists see new and different things when looking with familiar instruments in places they have looked before."

Thomas S. Kuhn again: "Nevertheless, paradigm changes do cause scientists to see the world of their research-engagement differently."

To be continued ...

Chapter 12

The Principle Applied to Alzheimer's Disease

In this chapter the Principle of Relations is applied to Alzheimer's disease. Since the cause of Alzheimer's is weakly understood, we must try alternative ideas.

First, an overview of the Alzheimer's disease:

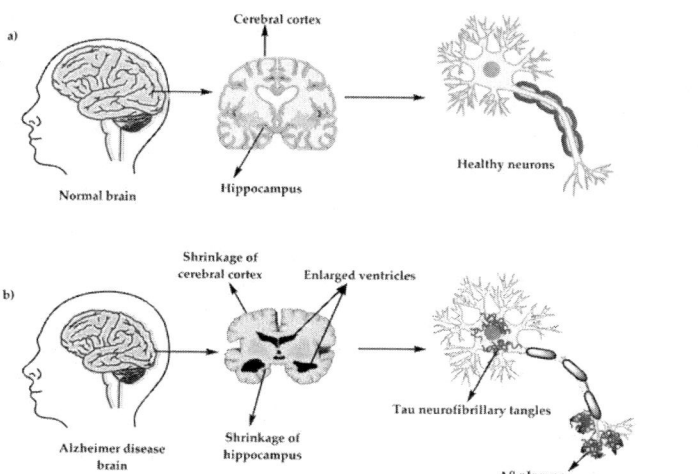

Source: imgurl:https://biologyease.com/wp-content/uploads/2021/04/Alzheimer-1024x756.png - Bing.

Figure 81. Alzheimer's disease and normal brain.

The physiological structure of the brain and neurons in (**a**) healthy brain and (**b**) Alzheimer's disease (AD) brain, from the source: Molecules | Free Full-Text | Comprehensive Review on Alzheimer's Disease: Causes and Treatment | HTML (mdpi.com)

Based on the postulate - Nothing exists in isolation; everything exists in relations - in combination with 1 and 2 above, then the principle is

$X = aRb,$

where X is inflammation and disease.

X = Alzheimer's disease. When microtubules are damaged and cannot perform intracellular transport of material, huge amount of amyloid beta will be crowded outside the cell and neurofibrillary tangles of tau proteins will occur inside the cell.

Based on the principle X = aRb, we find:

X = Alzheimer's disease, AD; i.e., AD = aRb. So when any network of tubules is damaged, it will cause AD.

The principle of relations claims that damaged flow dominates causing inflammation, while chronic inflammation causes disease. If damaged flows continue not being repaired, disease will be chronic, i.e., *when any flow is broken or damaged, there will be disorders and diseases, e.g., cancer, AV-block III, stroke, Alzheimer's and cardiac infarction.*

Then, the basic hypothesis for Alzheimer's disease will be: *When any network of tubules is damaged, it will cause Alzheimer's disease.*

The structure of aRb gives these alternative causes for Alzheimer's disease, i.e., damaged flows:

1. Gate failure of cell.
2. Microtubule damage.
3. Damaged flow contents.
4. Combination of 1-3.

We know that both amyloid beta and neurofibrillary tangles are involved in the disease. They are said to cause dysfunction within the brain's neuronal functions and their connectivity. When we use aRb to view the relationship between neuronal function and amyloid plaques/neurofibrillary tangles the causality will be the opposite, i.e., it is damaged flows between neurons that cause the symptoms of Alzheimer's.

First, the model of flow-block as a cause of Alzheimer's disease (AD):

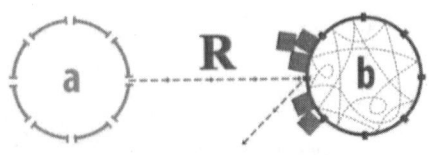

Figure 82. Model of Alzheimer's disease.

The Principle Applied to Alzheimer's Disease

When the gates are closed, no packages can either come into or leave the cell. Then the cell will be destroyed within, and outside it the packages will be crowded. Outside the cell, packages are crowded as senile plaques. Inside the cell, genetic disorder will occur. (It is not genetic disorder that causes and disrupts the cell's normal functioning.) The pictures below will show this:

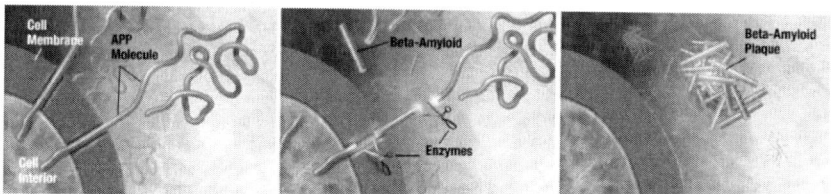

Source: New Hope for Fading Memories: Alzheimer's Disease | BioEd Online.

Figure 83. Alzheimer's cell.

So far, the facts, based on science, which correspond to the model of aRb, are:

1. Amyloid plaques outside the cell and neurofibrillary tangles inside the cell are involved.
2. Loss of neurons and synapses.
3. Inflammation.
4. Lower levels of Neurotrophic factors and the brain-derived neurotrophic factor, BDNF, (protein). (The activity of the neurotransmitter Alpha-7 nicotinic receptor (protein) is modulated by BDNF.)

In the representations below we can see numerous formations of plaque and tangles within the neuropil; to the left cerebral autopsy specimen of a patient diagnosed having Alzheimer disease. In the HE stain numerous plaque formations within the neuropil background are visible. (Credit: WIKIPEDIA, CC BY-SA 3.0 and to the right neuropil plaque - Bing).

Why do these plaques and tangles occur? How can we find the causes? How can we develop drugs to cure the disease?

If we do not have a basic principle and theory for understanding the human body, we will be drowned by all information given from the massive research efforts. So, by using the principle of relations and the formula $X = aRb$, we will have some guidance in our search for the causes of diseases.

By using the lens of this principle, we are mostly looking after the R_{1-n}, i.e., networks of relations consisting of flows and their content.

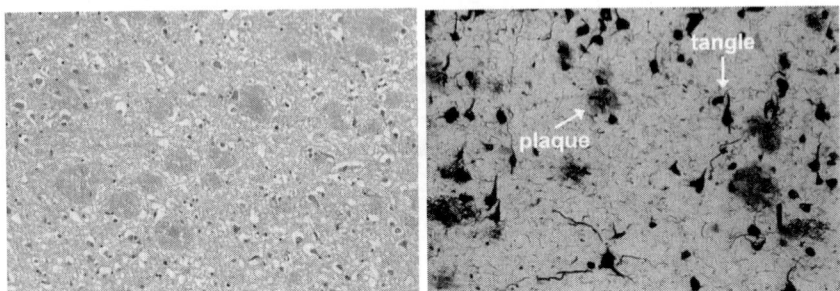

Figure 84.   **Figure 85.**

Source: Alzheimer's cell picture tangle plaque – Bildsökresultat (yahoo.com).

Figure 84 and 85. Plaque and tangle.

First, we focus on the concept and content of cytoskeleton, consisting of microtubules, microfilaments and intermediate filaments. The functions of the cytoskeleton are complex, but dealing with Alzheimer's disease, we focus on the dynamic network, i.e., the uptake of extracellular material (endocytosis), and organizing organelles. The cytoskeleton consists of filaments and microtubules, as the image below shows:

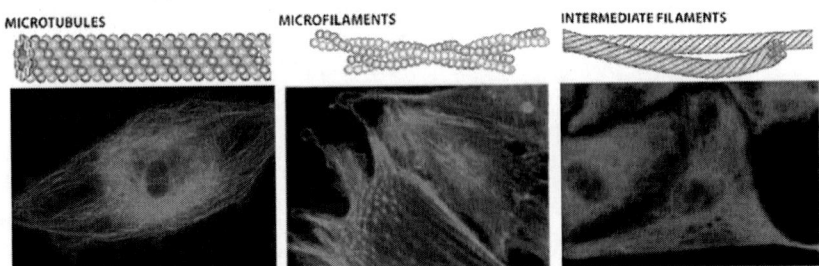

Source: Network of cytoskeletal filaments [5, 8] .... | Download Scientific Diagram (researchgate.net).

Figure 86. Tubules of the cell.

The cytoskeleton holds a nucleus enclosed within membranes and connects the cell nucleus with the membrane by means of with protein filaments.

The image below shows this, i.e., "human neural stem cells stained for Sox2, in green, and vimentin, in red. Vimentin is a type III intermediate filament (IF) protein":

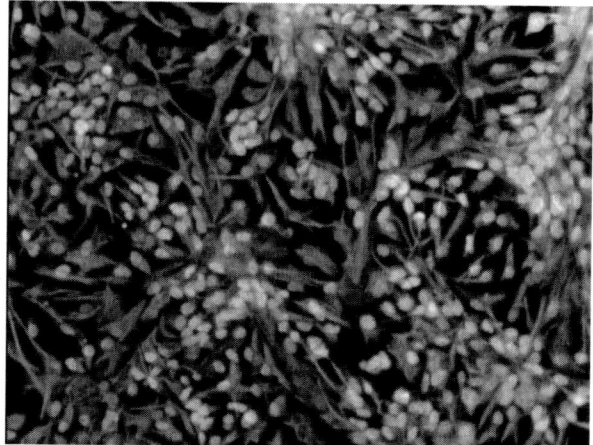

Source: Intermediate filament - Protein filament - Wikipedia.

Figure 87. Cytoskeleton of the cell.

Then, we find the cytoskeleton, which this image enables us to imagine:

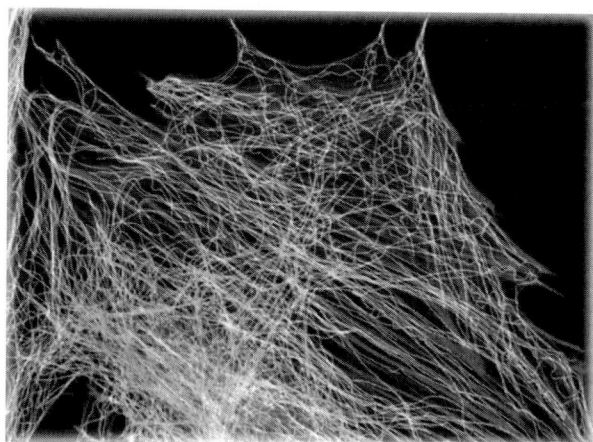

Source: Imaging the Cytoskeletal Network in 3T3 Cell Cultures | Olympus LS (olympus-lifescience.com.cn).

Figure 88. An alternative image of cytoskeleton.

The next image shows actin filaments in red and microtubules in green:

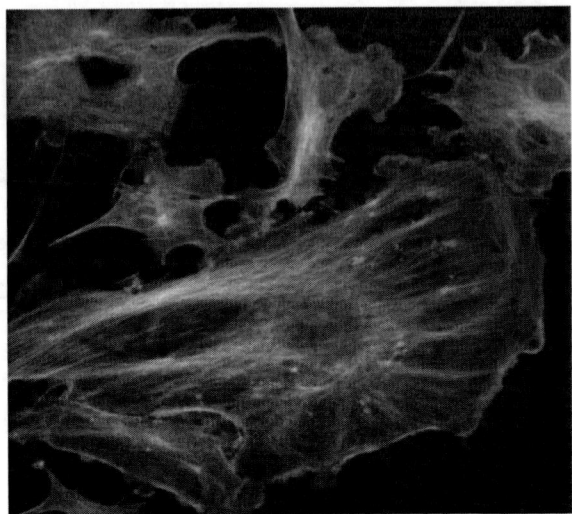

Source: Fluorescent Cells - Cytoskeleton - Wikipedia.

Figure 89. Filaments and microtubules.

The Logistic System and Its Flows within the Cell

The most important parts and concepts are the following:

1. Cytoskeleton
2. Microtubules
3. Microfilaments
4. Intermediate filaments
5. Axonal transport
6. Integrin

How is it possible to find which part of the logistic system causes diseases, since there are so many components to deal with?

Contemporary science mostly tries to find one cause and then develop drugs dealing with that part. But what if we have to find a combination of drugs, which can replace the entire function?

Is it possible to understand exactly which part is damaged and then direct drugs to that part only?

The Principle Applied to Alzheimer's Disease

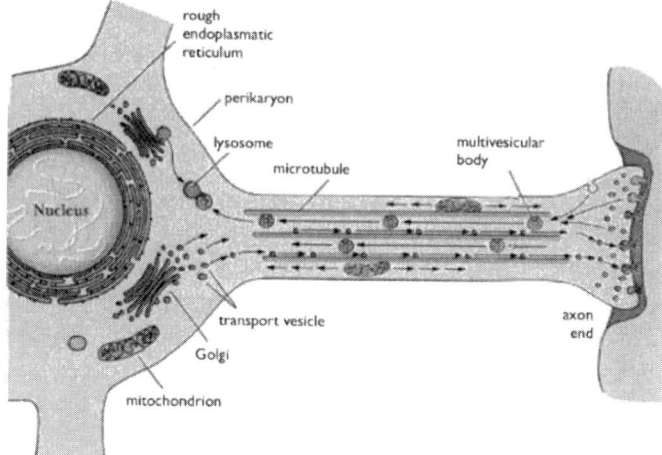

Source: Axon - Bing images.

Figure 90. Axon.

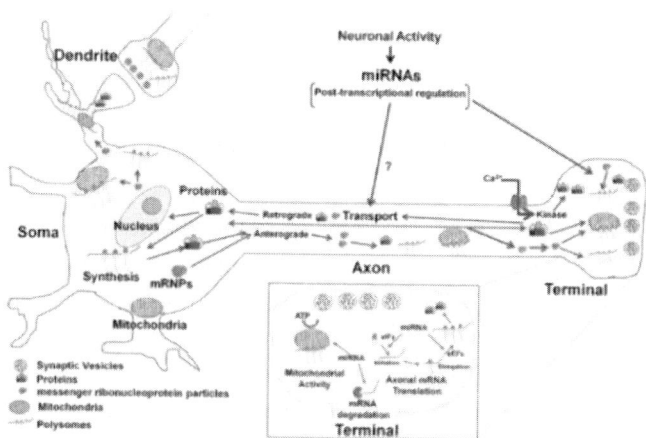

Source: axonal transport picture - Bing images.

Figure 91. An alternative image of axon.

We know that, in normal opening and closing of ion channels, the flow of ions passes through the membrane of a cell. Our first suspicion is that the gate will not open, for some reason. So, how can a gate recover from inactivity?

We will now focus on how damaged gates will affect the cytoskeleton's contact with the membrane and extracellular material.

How, then, to connect the cytoskeleton to extracellular material?

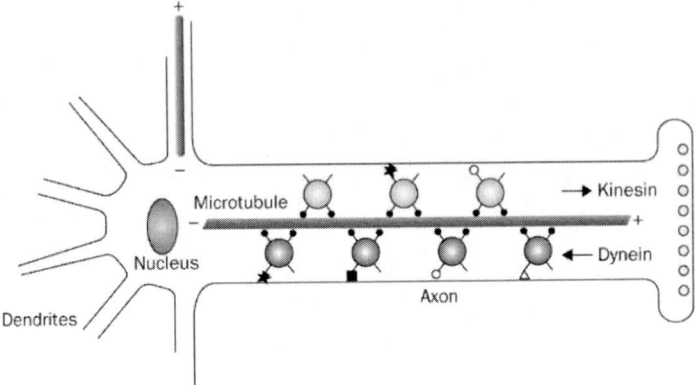

Source: axonal transport image - Bing images.

Figure 92. Axon transport image.

The receptor which connects the cytoskeleton to extracellular material is called *integrin*, which looks like a cyclical liaison. Integrins are receptors at the surface of the cell, fulfilling its mediation.

The image below shows how this is made, where E=extracellular space; I=intracellular space; P=plasma membrane, i.e., the function of transmembrane receptor:

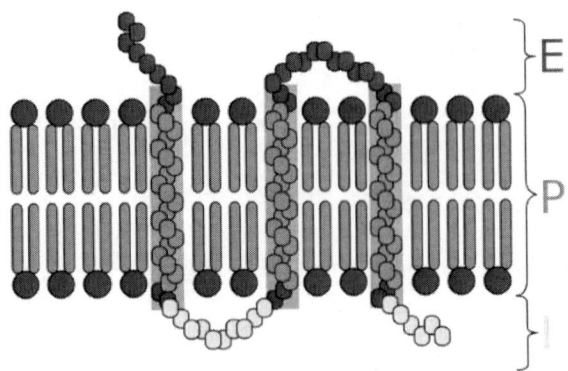

Source: Cell surface receptor - Wikipedia.

Figure 93. Integrin.

Integrin connects the cytoskeleton and the extracellular matrix. Based on aRb, damaged flows create Alzheimer's disease and if the integrin does not function it can be one possible cause for AD. Then, the figure below can be a guide giving us the first possible cause:

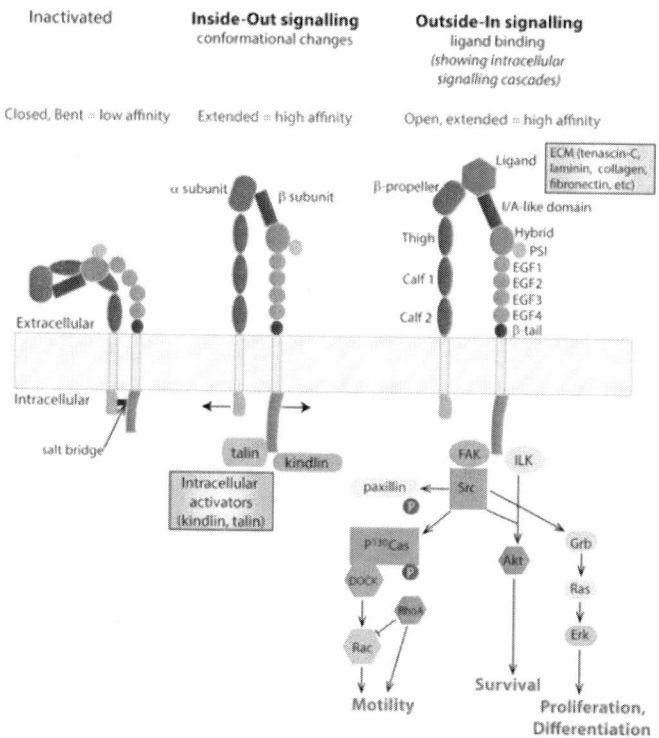

Source: Cells | Free Full-Text | Integrin Activation: Implications for Axon Regeneration | HTML (mdpi.com).

Figure 94. The complex integrin.

The figure describes the integrin Structure and Activation. "Activation of integrin heterodimers leads to intracellular signalling cascades and resulting processes such as cell motility, cell survival, cell differentiation, and neurite outgrowth. Schematic representing integrin conformations at the membrane including changes that occur with 'Inside–Out signalling' and 'Outside–In signalling'. An inactivated integrin heterodimer exists with a closed and bent conformation (extracellularly) stabilised by a cytoplasmic salt bridge. This conformation has a very low ligand binding affinity. With Inside–Out signalling, intracellular activators (such as kindlin and talin) bind the β subunit cytoplasmically and interact/destabilise the salt bridge, leading to an open and extended (active) conformation with increased ligand binding affinity. With Outside–In signalling, binding of a ligand (ECM molecules such as laminin, fibronectin, or tenascin) extracellularly occurs as a result of integrin activation leading to a conformational change to an open and extended (active) conformation with high ligand binding affinity. Individual names of the extracellular domain components have been shown in the Outside–In signalling example for simplicity, with further explanation in the main text." (Source: Cells | Free Full-Text | Integrin Activation: Implications for Axon Regeneration | HTML (mdpi.com)).

In the article *Integrin Activation: Implications for Axon Regeneration*, the authors Menghon Cheah and Melissa R. Andrews also conclude that "As integrins are essential for the proper functioning of a normal and healthy nervous system, translational researchers in the field of axon regeneration have been trying to harvest the use of integrins following a central nervous system (CNS) injury, such as spinal cord injury, in order to recapitulate a developmental growth state that could enhance regenerative growth."

But, how can we find out the function of an integrin, when it is large, complex and linked to many sugar trees? (Integrin - Wikipedia)

Even after many years of research and hundreds of papers, it is not possible to find the structure of integrins.

One attempt is based on this model, made by Richard O. Hynes. (PII: S0092-8674(02)00971-6 (cell.com).

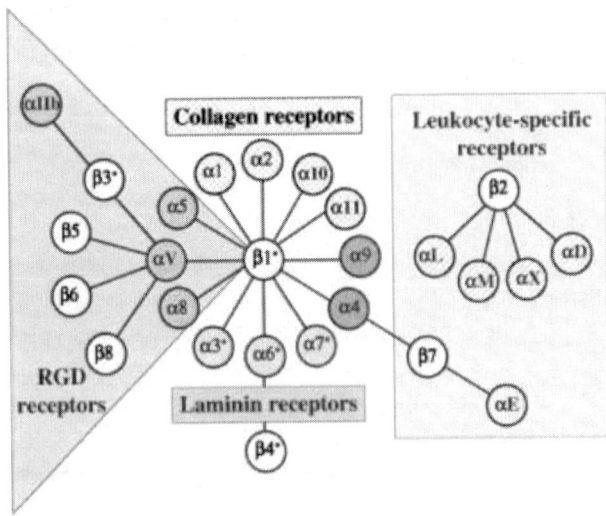

Figure 95. Integrin interpretation.

We are told that "integrins are αβ heterodimes; each subunit crosses the membrane once, with most of each polypeptide (>1600 amino acids in total) in the extracellular space and two short cytoplasmic domains (20-50 amino acids). ..."

Then, is the answer to the questions of the cause of AD damaged integrin? And then, how can reparation of integrins cure AD?

It is obvious that some transformation will fulfil the function of transportation of molecules, but it is not certain that integrin is the answer. So we might as well, based on the principle of relations, create an alternative solution: as told before the name is *transformer*. The shape of a transformer, looking like a paddle wheel, will differ depending on where it is located. The image below might stimulate our imagination (the size will be measured in nanometres, approximately 50-200 nm), where each number can accept only one specific particle from a molecule, e.g., H, N, P, C and O, at the left side, and then a new molecule will occur, e.g., $C_{10}H_{16}N_5O_{13}P_3$, at the right side:

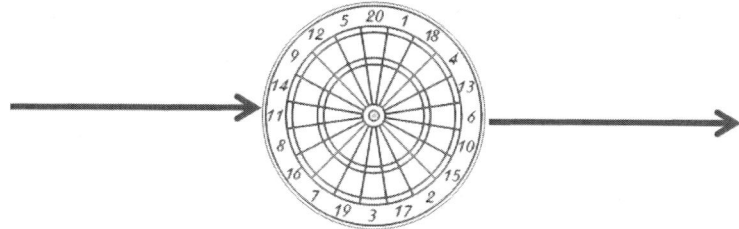

Figure 96. The Transformer.

Throughout reality the Transformer functions by the same principal mechanism, e.g., the Earth, the Sun, the Moon, the human body, galaxies, black holes, organs and cells in the human body.

Now, let's deal with a possible drug curing AD, called a manifold drug.

A Manifold Drug for Alzheimer'S Disease

How can we find drugs for Alzheimer's disease?

In this Chapter a new method for finding drugs is proposed. We have seen how many factors can be the cause of AD, so we have to create a manifold drug, i.e., a combination of integrin protein, kinesin, dynein and others.

Contemporary science often uses this model for clarifying status in dealing with drugs for Alzheimer's disease:

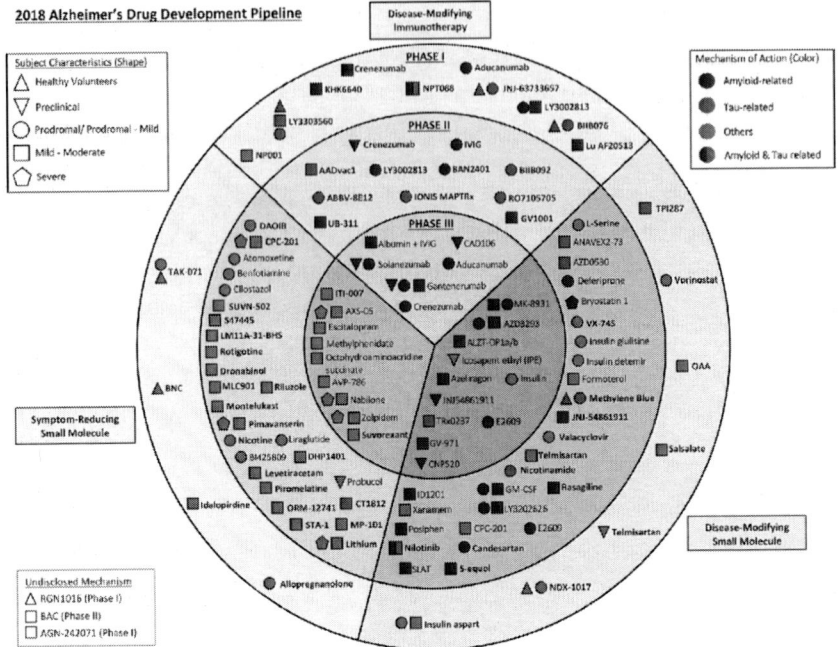

Source: alzheimer's drugs in clinical trials - Sök (bing.com).

Figure 97. Overview of Alzheimer's drugs.

This model shows how different approaches try to handle inflammation and targeting the tau protein tangles which are linked to and occur in Alzheimer's disease, but the cause of AD is still not yet known, so drugs cannot successfully be developed.

We have to test another angle finding medicine for AD. If we focus on multifactorial drugs, then the content of the medicine might be:

- Kindlin-3, which has a role in the function of integrin activation
- Talin
- Ligand
- Salt bridge

Kindlin-3 is also known as FERM3. Below in the figure we find how it works out dealing with the integrin (Source: The kindlin family: functions,

The Principle Applied to Alzheimer's Disease 119

signaling properties and implications for human disease | Journal of Cell Science | The Company of Biologists):

The COOH represents the carboxyl group, and the most common organic acids are organic carboxylic acids.

Talin activation and membrane recruitment, by engaging:

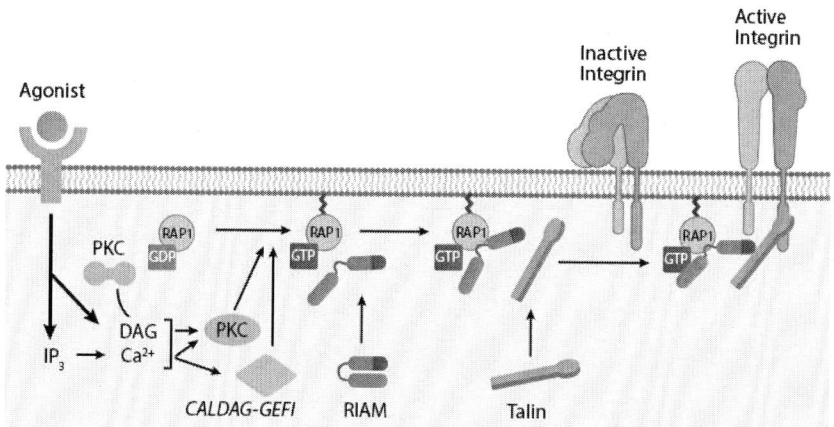

Source: imgurl:https://www.mechanobio.info/wp-content/uploads/2017/06/Talin-Recruitment-to-Membrane.jpg - Bing.

Figure 98. Membrane functionality.

Below is a cobalt complex $HCo(CO)_4$ with five ligands:

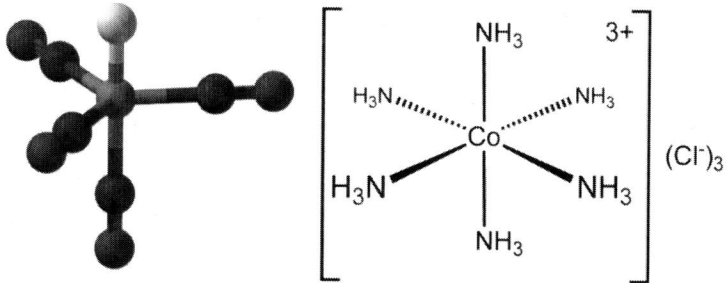

Source: imgurl:https://upload.wikimedia.org/wikipedia/commons/thumb/f/fd/CoA6Cl3.png/400px-CoA6Cl3.png - Bing.

Figure 99. Cobalt.

The figure below is an example of a salt bridge between acids glutamic acid and lysine.

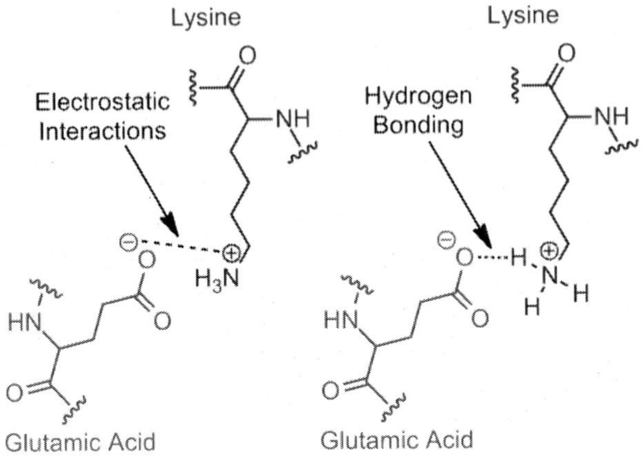

Source: imgurl:https://upload.wikimedia.org/wikipedia/commons/thumb/b/b4/Next
_Revisit_Glutamic_Acid_Lysine_salt_bridge.png/450px-Next_Revisit_
Glutamic_Acid_Lysine_salt_bridge.png - Bing.
Source: Next Revisit Glutamic Acid Lysine salt bridge - Salt bridge (protein and supramolecular) - Wikipedia.

Figure 100. Salt bridge.

How, Then, Can We Create a Manifold Drug and Treatment for AD?

Starting with molecules and their atoms, then we create a new molecule as drug for AD.

The atoms and the molecules are the following:

1. Glutamic acid using the atoms C, H, N, O and its formula is $C_5H_9NO_4$
2. Ligands using the atoms H, C, O, o and its formula is $HCo(CO)_4$
3. Lysine uses the atoms N, H and its formula is $-NH_3^+$
4. The salt bridge uses the atoms H, O, N, R and its formula and function can be seen in these two figures, connecting two halves of the molecular capsule:

The Principle Applied to Alzheimer's Disease

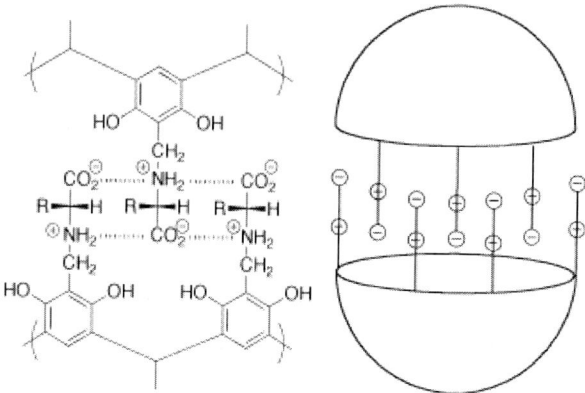

Source: image. Molecular capsule – Bildsökresultat (yahoo.com).

Figure 101. Molecular capsule.

It seems obvious that the understanding of how mass moves in the human body is not fully understood. Then we have two choices dealing with drugs and treatment for AD:

1. By a combination of atoms and molecules, based on what has been told above, create the drug.
2. Accept one superior aRb and by its activation repair the cell.

We have to find the dominant and superior aRb, which dictates the process. We must implement a system for fulfilling flows of atoms and molecules. The flow of C – H – N – O – H – C - O – N – H – H must be reassured.

Now we have to find out how to organize this chain C – H – N – O – H – C - O – N – H – H.

Then we have to produce the molecule and find out how to inject it in the human body, i.e., how to put it in to the brain.

This is a demanding iterative process engaging hundreds of scientists and thousands of lab tests and clinical trials before the molecule becomes a drug seen as a masterpiece.

To be continued ...

Chapter 13

The Principle Applied to Diseases of Kidney, Heart, ADHD, Mental Illness and the Human Conciousness

The Principle Applied to the Kidney

Kidney filtration diseases occur when the flow of packages is damaged.

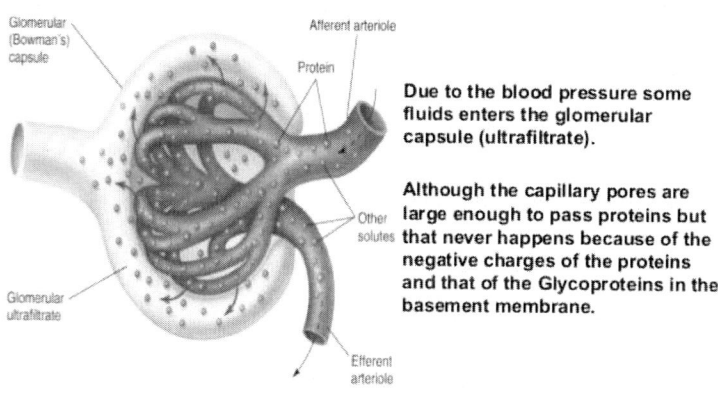

Source: picture Glomerular ultrafiltrate – Bildsökresultat (yahoo.com).

Figure 102. Glomerular ultrafiltrate.

The Principle Applied to the Heart

The disease AV-block III occurs when the flow of packages is damaged.
    Normally, the pathway of the heart's electrical system has this structure, (Atrioventricular block - Wikipedia):

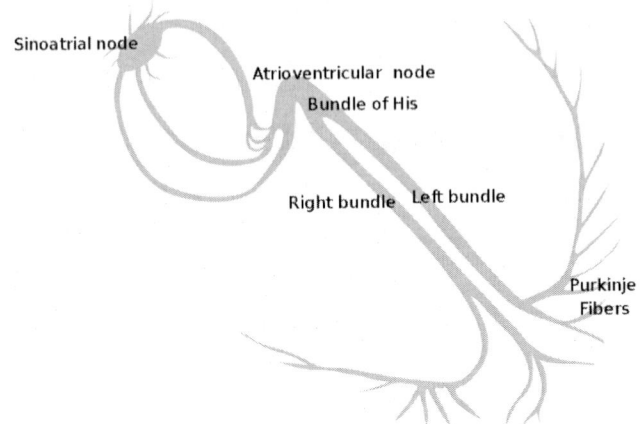

Source: Nodes of the heart – Bildsökresultat (yahoo.com).

Figure 103. Nodes of the heart.

Third-Degree Heart Block, as shown below, (119ced8b726f847aa 2d20018c5561752.jpg (473×345) (pinimg.com):

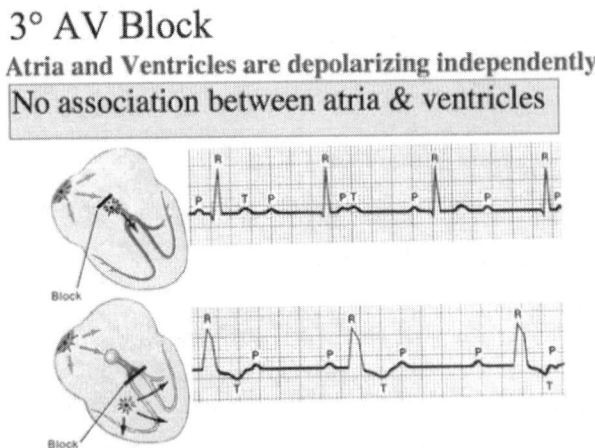

Source: av-block heart – Bildsökresultat (yahoo.com).

Figure 104. AV Block III.

Now we have to understand how the system of impulses between the SA node and the AV node functions. Again we start with the concept tubules and their content.

Tubules are organized in a complex network, i.e., connecting cells within the heart and transport ions.

The Principle Applied to ADHD

ADHD, Attention-Deficit/Hyperactivity Disorder, means difficulties in concentration and control of activities and impulses.

Based on aRb it is the society and the relations in the societal network that cause ADHD, via damage in the neurotransmitter system of the brain. As for now, we understand that flows of packages are essential for normal functioning in any system and when flows of packages of dopamine and norepinephrine in the pathways of the brain are damaged, ADHD will occur. To some extent there are similarities between the network structure of relations for the individual human being, the network structure of relations for the neurotransmitter system in the brain and the structure of the human psyche. This is based on the flow of packages between the three levels, thus causing ADHD, as shown in the figure below:

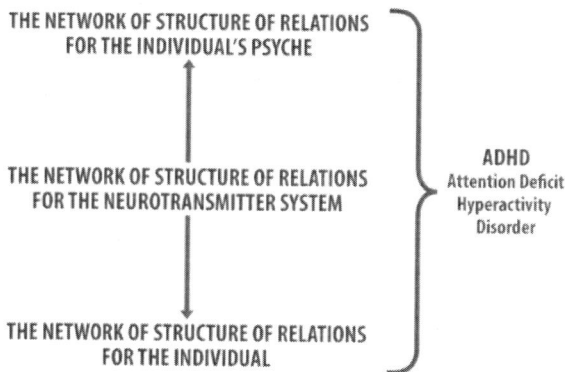

Figure 105. ADHD.

ADHD is increasing in countries such as the USA: one report shows an increase of over 40% over a period of eight years, from 2003 to 2011; and there are indications of increase in most parts of the world. Based on aRb, ADHD gives an indication that society in all its complexity must focus on dealing with ADHD.

Modern society has some new phenomena such as ADHD, burn-out, Alzheimer's, ADD, DAMP, dementia and similar diseases.

The major challenge is to overcome these diseases, since it seems that they all are a consequence of a dysfunctional society and dysfunctional networks.

The Principle Applied to Human Consciousness and Psyche

Based on aRb, consciousness is the result of the flow of packages which occur from objects outside the human, but it can also occur from objects inside the human, such as body pain and dreams. These packages constitute the memory, which is the consequence of the same molecular movements over and over again, until there is a pattern in the brain, which will be triggered by the same stimuli of objects. The structure and pattern of the memory is a continuous flow of packages. It will only change by the arrival of new packages, depending on how strongly the pattern has been established. In the worst case, when a mental disorder has come up, it is possible to make the brain healthy again by using an intense flow of alternative packages.

Consciousness is then a combination of memory patterns of flows of packages and the flow of packages from outside objects, i.e., consciousness is a flow of thoughts in real time.

The structure of the human psyche, b, is affected by R, from a. When R is damaged, the psyche will develop diseases such as schizophrenia or suicidal behaviour.

Isolation and desolation, i.e., damaged R, is often the reason for diseases of the psyche, based on the postulate.

To fully understand the content in R between a and b in a social network is not easy. However there are some obvious contents, such as food logistics, heating of the house, water supply, clothes and furniture. All that is needed on a daily basis. When it comes to feelings, emotions and words like love, the content, in concrete concepts, is not that easy to understand. However there is a chemistry of love, where testosterone and oestrogen, dopamine and serotonin are involved, combined with our sense of smell. That is why we need to start at the level of the consequences of a lack of R in these relations.

We know from the research of the sociologist Emile Durkheim and his book *Suicide*, that in Protestant countries the rate of suicide is higher than in Catholic countries due to the fact that in Protestant countries people are more individual with fewer relations to other people. It is not psychological diseases that are the causes; it is isolation, desolation and loneliness. In Sweden 1.500 persons, mostly men, commit suicide every year.

We know, based on science, that solitude and loneliness, especially for men, are the reason not only for suicide, but also for bad health and early death. It can be compared with smoking too much or drinking too much, which is a frequent combination for solitary and isolated men, since it is mostly men who will be affected. Men in solitude die much earlier than married men.

Loneliness and isolation, which is damaged R, increase the risks for both mental health and physical health, such as high blood pressure and heart problems, especially for older people. New-born children can in the worst case die without physical contact. Loneliness kills. Loneliness predicts depression, suicide, cancer, cardiovascular diseases, stroke, risk of dementia, high cholesterol; it is in fact a life-threating condition.

Everyone needs love and care in solid relations. If the closest relations are dysfunctional with social isolation, especially from an absent and charismatic father, the risk of schizophrenia will increase. How the damaged relation R will affect a child is rather well known, however it has to be explored again based on aRb.

Furthermore, the individual's relations in the family, with relatives and friends, are also affected by the surrounding society, which in turn is dependent on national and international relations.

It is family and friends who make us happy; to be famous and to have riches and wealth, which instead can lead to isolation and loneliness, do not make us happy. What a paradox!

To maintain good health, both mentally and physically, loneliness and isolation must be conquered. To be part of a network of people will bring us a happy, healthy and long life.

We need to explore this table in detail:

The individual's psyche	Systems, parts and elements	Relations	Systems, parts and elements	Broken relation	Disorder disease	Repair of relation
Flow	a Structure of a	Content of Packages	b Structure of b	Isolation	Suicide Early death	

Please accept this too short text, just see it as a starting point.
So ...
To be continued ...

Chapter 14

A Medical Tool for Diagnosis and Treatment by Cell Transplants in Order to Restore Damaged Flows

As yet, this is the most difficult and demanding part, but to start the journey, let's make an attempt.

Two examples of diagnosis with a tool of R, then correcting R:

1. A pacemaker corrects the beating of the heart and overcomes AV-block III.
2. A "brain maker" corrects the relation between cells in the brain and makes them work normally (not yet invented).
3. Etc.

Establish a cross–organic team within fields such as brain, heart, kidney, lever, neurology etc in order to develop a tool for securing diagnosis and curing. This team will handle existing knowledge.

The team will direct an operational team, which will create a computer-based software. The program can handle information concerning diseases and symptoms in order to make a correct diagnosis and ordinate the right medicine and treatment for a specific disease. It shall guide a doctor to understand complications with different medicines in relation to a specific disease. If a patient has high blood pressure, weak kidneys and AV-block 3 on the heart, what will then happen? (Fainting when driving a car at full speed, which is dangerous)

The tool will help a single doctor to make the best diagnosis and treatment for a single patient. If the treatment is proposed to be Metoprolol, then the doctor put this information into the computer program and he will get an answer, maybe that the combination will lead to fainting or even worse to death.

The next step is to focus on diagnosis and treatment based on the principle of relations.

So far, transplantation has been done with organs. Now, there are too few donors for most organs, so we need to find new ways of repairing damaged organs.

There are three levels to focus on:

1. Organs
2. Cells
3. Molecules

We must now find a method for cell transplantation of damaged flow in the body.

If we can find a generic method to transplant cells to different organs in the body, there might be a chance to cure some diseases. Here I will focus on three applications:

1. Internodal Pathway in the heart.
2. The kidney filtration mechanism.
3. Cancer

Different cells have different functions, but the method of transplantation can be the same.

Questions:

1. How to transplant a cell or a group of cells?
2. How to transplant a kidney cell?
3. How to transplant an internodal pathway cell?

Preliminary reflections:

1. We will use the same instrument as when a plug is removed in the heart's coronal vessel, but instead in the front, there will be a nippers or tongs. With this instrument we will get the cells from a donor.
2. The next step is, with the same instrument, where the front has an opener that will put the cell in place. The cell is placed in the injured kidney or in the damaged internodal pathway in the heart or into the cancer area.

Further questions:

1. How can we reduce the risk of rejection?
2. How will the cells be integrated in the organ?

Preliminary reflections:

1. The immune response is well known in science. It is complex when it comes to graft rejection. We need to be advised from skilled operators.
2. "Steroid-free treatment regimen" is well known in science.

There are now some discussions as to whether the cell transplantation will consist of stem cell repairing organs or whether mature cells can repair cells and organs.

For inspiration, see link below about Susan Lim: https://www.youtube.com/watch?v=PJtS2YH4Ny0

Susan Lim is talking about "From organ transplantation to cell transplantation": those stem cells can repair organs.

Benjamin Humphreys, PhD, a Harvard Medical School assistant professor was suspicious and he suggested kidney cells themselves have capacity to divide after injury. In a test the team around him found that mature cells, in mice, showed that the cells multiply several times to help repair the kidney.

Kidney Repair May Not Require Stem Cells

Harvard Stem Cell Institute (HSCI) researchers have a new model for how the kidney repairs itself, a model that adds to a growing body of evidence that mature cells are far more plastic than had previously been imagined.

"After injury, mature kidney cells dedifferentiate into more primordial versions of themselves, and then differentiate into the cell types needing replacement in the damaged tissue. This finding conflicts with a previously held theory that the kidney has scattered stem cell populations that respond to injury. The research appears online today in *PNAS Early Edition*.

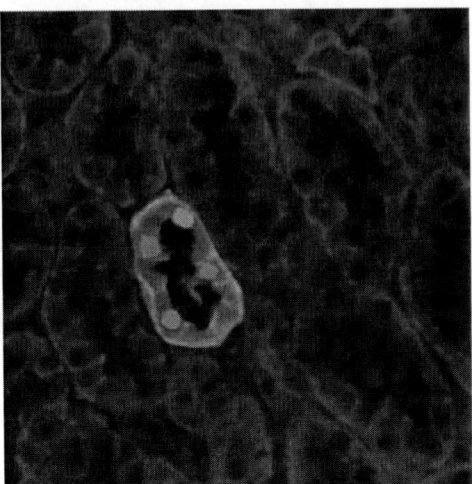

Source: Stem cell – Bildsökresultat (yahoo.com).

Figure 106. Stem cell.

HSCI Kidney Disease Program Leader Benjamin Humphreys, MD, PhD, a Harvard Medical School assistant professor at Brigham and Women's Hospital, was suspicious of the kidney stem cell repair model because his previous work suggested that all kidney cells have the capacity to divide after injury. He and his colleagues decided to test conventional wisdom by genetically tagging mature kidney cells in mice that do not express stem cell markers; the hypothesis being that the mature cells should do nothing or die after injury. The results showed that not only do these fully differentiated cells multiply, but *they can multiply several times as they help to repair the kidney.*"[1]

"What was really interesting is when we looked at the appearance and expression patterns of these differentiated cells, we found that they expressed the exact same 'stem cell markers' that these other groups claimed to find in their stem cell populations," said Humphreys. "And so, if a differentiated cell is able to express a 'stem cell marker' after injury, then what our work shows is that that's an injury marker—it doesn't define a stem cell."

This new interpretation of kidney repair suggests a model by which cells reprogram themselves; similar to the way mature cells can be chemically manipulated to revert to an induced pluripotent state. The research echoes a study published last month by HSCI Principal Faculty member David Breault, MD, PhD, who showed that cells in the adrenal glands also regenerate by means of natural lineage conversion.

A Medical Tool for Diagnosis and Treatment by Cell Transplants ...   133

"One has to remember that not every organ necessarily is endowed with clear and well-defined stem cell populations, like the intestines or the skin," Humphreys explained. "I'm not saying that kidney stem cells don't exist, but in tissues where cell division is very slow during homeostasis, there may not have been an evolutionary pressure for stem cell mechanisms of repair."

"He plans to apply his kidney repair discovery to define new therapeutic targets in acute kidney injury. The goal would be to find drugs that accelerate the process of dedifferentiation and proliferation of mature kidney cells in response to injury, as well as slow down pathways that impair healing or lead to scar tissue formation."

However, there might be a chance to transplant a kidney cell in order to restore the filtration function in injured kidneys.

So, how to move forward?

Some Pictures to Engage the Imagination

When we find a damaged flow and the reason for it, we can repair the injury by using a nipper tool, which will put in place a new component and take away the damaged component.

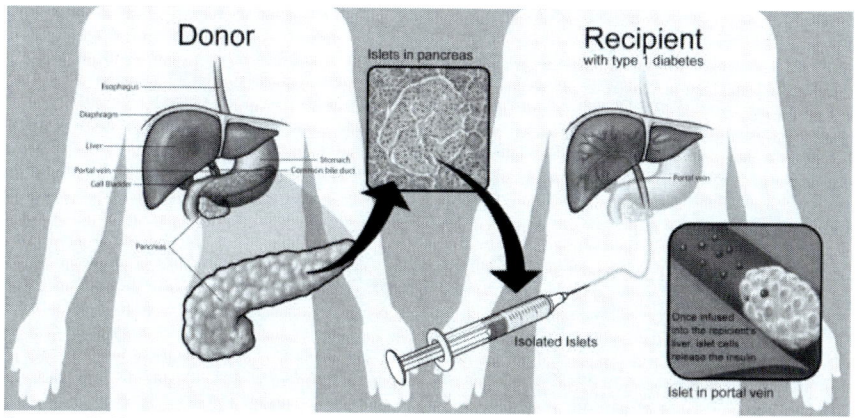

Source: Cell transplant pictures – Bildsökresultat (yahoo.com).

Figure 107. Cell transplant.

The Same Is Valid for the Kidney

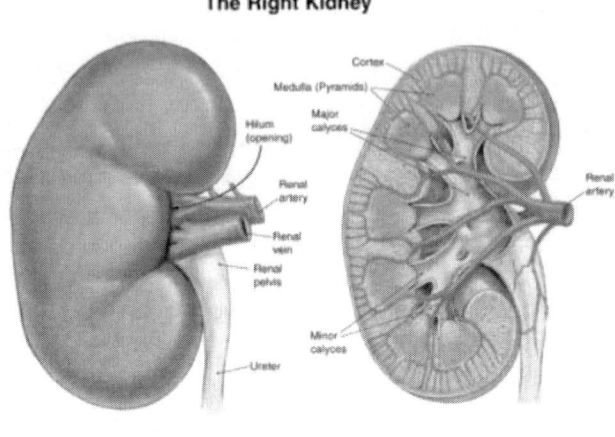

Source: Picture Kidney – Bildsökresultat (Yahoo.Com).

Figure 108. Kidney.

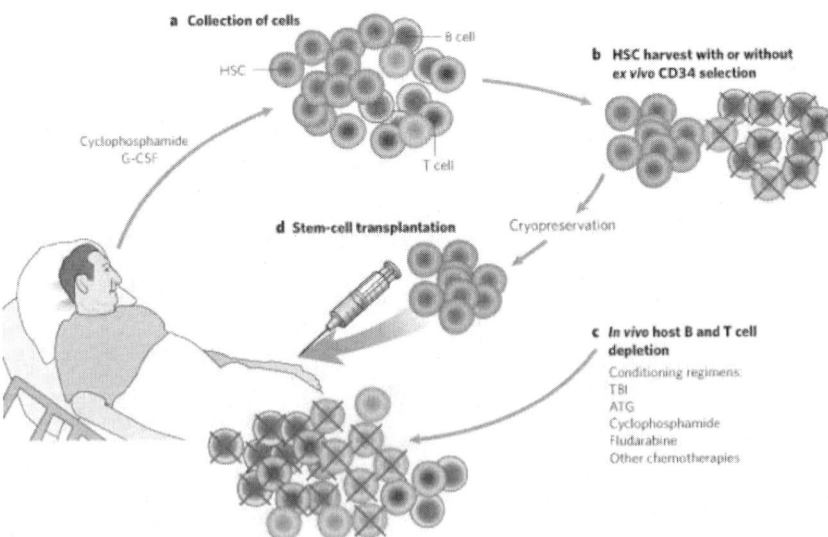

Source: Cell transplant pictures – Bildsökresultat (yahoo.com).

Figure 109. Cell transplantation.

Internodal Pathways, Transmitting Impulse from SA Node to AV Node

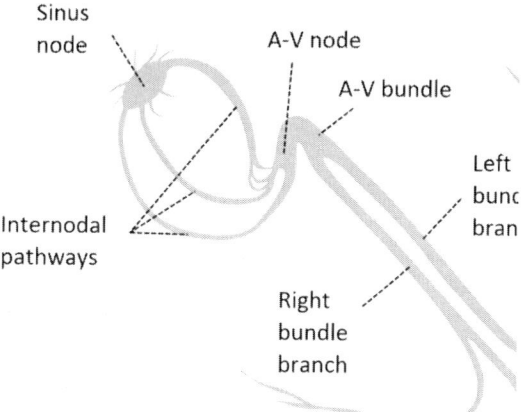

Source: Internodal pathways pictures – Bildsökresultat (yahoo.com).

Figure 110. Internodal pathways.

How Cancer Cell Can Be Invaded by Normal Cell via Transplantation

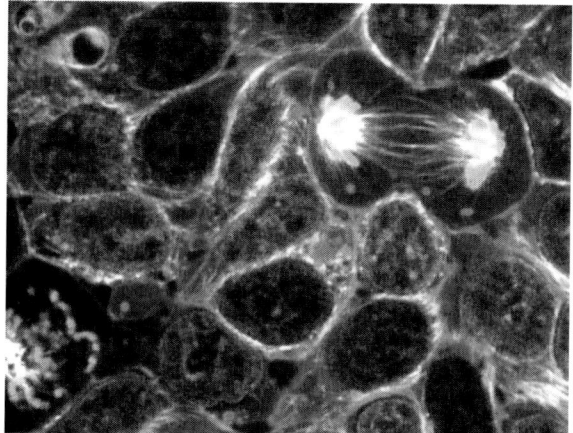

Source: Cancer intervention pictures – Bildsökresultat (yahoo.com).

Figure 111. Cancer intervention.

Now, we have to find those cells to be transplanted to the kidney and the heart.

How to Move Forward

Team for steering:
Team for operation:
Finance:
Table of analysis:

Analysis	Symptoms	Fever	Fainting
Organs:			
Heart			
Kidney			
Etc.			

Of course, to be continued ...

Chapter 15

Two Different Theories Dealing with the Human Body

The Paradigm of the Human Body - P_H - as it shows up today in the contemporary science of medicine, is based on these statements, concepts and theories:

1. The science of the human body is built on the analogy with a house: the sum of different parts constitutes a human body.
2. Physiology as science uses concepts based on concepts from the mechanical, physical, bioelectrical and biochemical sciences, in the study both of human organs and of the cells of which they are composed.
3. The human body is made up of certain elements.
4. The focus is on organs and systems.
5. Most research is done on subsystems.

The Principle of Relations, P_R, is based on these statements regarding the human body:

1. The human body is a system of relations consisting of flows of packages.
2. $S_H = (aRb)^{-\infty} = S_i R_1 S_m R_2 S_c \; R_3 S_l R_4 S_r R_5 S_d R_6 S_u R_7 S_{re} R_8 S_n R_9 S_e \; R_{10} S_s.$
3. There is a system of hierarchical systems between all aRb.
4. Diagnosis can be made by an analysis of R, as a tool, which can then correct R, and so prevent, cure and reduce disease.

:

Human body	Systems, parts and elements		Relations	Systems, parts and elements		Broken relation	Disorder/disease	Repair of relation
	a	Structure of a	Content of Packages	b	Structure of b			
Flow Blood	oxygen food		bind to hemaglobin blood plasma via blood vessels	cells cells				
Lymph	lymph nodes		blood without red blood cells via lymph vessels	lymph nodes				
Blood Urine	blood plasma		proteins via vesicles Via channel systems nephrons are connected to ureter	molecule urinary bladder				
Blood	kidney		via blood fat step ...	kidney		flow-block at the kidney will develop to surgical cyst and at the end stop functioning high blood pressure		
Electrical signals in the heart	electrical conduction system of the heart				impulses generated from SA-node stimulate the cardiac muscle	AV-block III	At the end death	Pacemaker or gate repairing of the ion channel
	cell		glucose supply	brain		gating failed and no glucose	Alzheimer's	
	cell			species				
	organs			DNA				
	species			DNA				
	cell			DNA				
	cell			organ				
	molecule			organ				
	cell	gating	glucose	cells		no glucose to cells and a lot glucose to cancer cells, due to failed gating	cancer	
							Schizophrenia stroke heart attack	
	cell					changes in the various pathways increase glucose metabolism	cancer	

Figure 112. Overview of the human body.

P_R has these consequences:

1. When any R in S_H is broken, there will be a disease such as cancer, high creatinine, AV-block III ...
2. When any R is broken, disorder and damage will occur.
3. There is a need for a survey and a map of all R_{1-n} in the human body.
4. Now, tools can be created that will influence broken R, in order to repair, prevent and reduce diseases.
5. The Principle of Relations has already been analysed when it comes to the transport system in cells. Cells organize the route of the packages, P_{1-n}, and how the packages of molecules in vesicles find their destinations and deliver the content. This mechanism, R, will cause diseases when it is disordered. Research based on correlation can now be changed to research based on relations. Most research today investigates how phenomena exist at the same time, where one phenomenon is the cause of the second phenomenon, e.g., how smoking cause's lung cancer and how bacteria cause inflammation.

Now we can start up summarizing all relations and diseases by the table shown in Figure 112.

Conclusion

The accepted opinion is that physics is the most fundamental science and that medicine, chemistry and other disciplines are built on it.

I am not sure this is the final answer and I will argue that, most likely, the fundament and foundation of science is based not on different matters/materials as in physics, but on the logic of principles, dealing with the behaviour of the objects in all sciences, i.e., *how the behaviour of the physical reality occurs, regardless of its content.*

Once we define the concepts *physical* and *reality* to mean the same object; i.e., in saying "reality" we are also saying "physical," they are just two concepts denoting the same - "thing" - then concepts and postulates dealing with the physics do not have implications for other disciplines, e.g., the science of medicine, since by this definition medicine deals with reality and might as well be the starting point for all sciences, by launching this new principle – as shown in this paper.

Today the science of medicine is mostly based on two postulates:

1. Causal reasoning, i.e., to make sense of cause and effect.
2. The human body is controlled by the laws of physics.

The new postulate for medicine is:

1. *Nothing exists in isolation, i.e., everything exists in relations.*

This postulate is valid for scientific objects as well as for human sciences, i.e., the postulate is at the most fundamental level, before we even think of science and humans; this is valid for all objects and all beings.

However, let us first investigate postulates 1 and 2.

1. When it comes to causal reasoning, i.e., to make sense of cause and effect, we know that the three causes of diseases are injury, toxicity and deficiency. We also know quite well which components causes diseases, e.g., processed food, physical and emotional stress, electromagnetic radiation, lack of calories and water, lack of rest, lack of fresh air, lack of sun and lack of love.

However, how to describe the detailed and concrete chain of occurrences linking these components to the diseases? How and in what way does a cause generate an effect?
2. The human body is controlled by the laws of physics. Over time we must expect and accept that the laws of physics will be changed, so the science of medicine should not rely too much on them. Physics still has unsolved questions to deal with, e.g., how to unite the theory of general relativity and theories of quantum. So the postulates which rely on physics are not, over time, stable enough for medicine to have as a prerequisite. A new paradigm of physics will come, as it always has done.

Sometimes postulates 1 and 2 are confusing, stating that a force, a causal power, is the cause of an effect, e.g., a disease. Force is a concept used in physics, e.g., a body in rest needs some the force to go into motion, and it is a force that causes a unit to change its motion.

Based on statistics, such as Austin Bradford Hill's nine criteria, we identify smoking as the cause and lung cancer its effect. This is a causal relationship, but, again, *how to describe the chain of cause and effect in concrete terms*?

This mechanical view finds nature as a system of causes and effects in space and time[2]. But this view restricts our mind and, since we must look further, it can also damage our thinking. This is understandable, but it will damage our opportunities to understand more of the reality of medicine and the human body.

Let us now turn to postulate 3 and how it might explain diseases and how that would affect medicine as a science.

First, we need to define some important concepts as below. Then we will have a platform for understanding the human body from a new perspective, even if this is obvious for most physicians, i.e., nothing exists in isolation, not a part, not a system; everything is connected to continuous flows and impacts between all parts and all systems. Consequently all cells and organs in the human body receive and deliver flows of packages in and out of cells and organs each microsecond; the human body also receives and delivers flows of packages outside of the body, e.g., eating, breathing, working, loving and socializing.

Based on the postulate, the fundamental concepts and the fundamental equations behind the laws of relations will be the following:

Conclusion

The concept relation relates to reality by showing that there are relations between all parts in the Universe, where:

1. **a, b, c** ... are any system, subsystem, unit or part in any field of the Universe, e.g., suns, planets, moons, galaxies, atoms, molecules, cells, organs and species.
2. The relation, **R,** is a flow (wave) of packages, p_{1-n}, e.g., quarks, protons, neutrons, electrons, photons, proteins, fats, polysaccharides, between a, b, c ... in any field of the Universe.

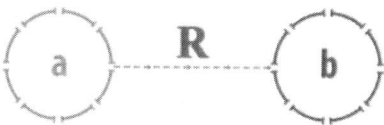

Figure 113. The basic model of relations.

Based on the postulate - *nothing exists in isolation, i.e., everything exists in relations* – in combination with 1 and 2 above, the principle is

X = aRb

The principle of relations claims that between all systems and between all parts of any system, S, there is a continuous flow of packages p_{1-n}, i.e., in aRb, $R = p_{1-n}$, and the formula is

S = ap_{1-n}b

S is a complex of relations between all parts and elements in the system, i.e., the a, b, and c are complicated systems, which send and/or receive flows of packages, i.e., p_{1-n}

$$R = \sum p_{1-n} = p_1 + p_2 + p_3 \ldots p_n$$

The big challenge is now to identify all the *p* in all relations and to identify, certainly and concretely, the logic of

$$S_1 = (a_1R_1b_1)\ R_2\ (a_2R_3b_2) \ldots$$

The Principle of Relations is based on these statements:

1. There cannot be any fixed atomic facts and elementary propositions.
2. There are no values which are true or false, but only true or false at a certain point of time.
3. Based on the postulate, the concepts of conjunction, disjunction, implication, negation and plus are not valid. Nature is not based on the logic of conjunction, negation and implication; it is based on the logic of relations.

This is the model of the Human Body, based on the alternative postulate, *nothing exists in isolation, and everything exists in relations:*

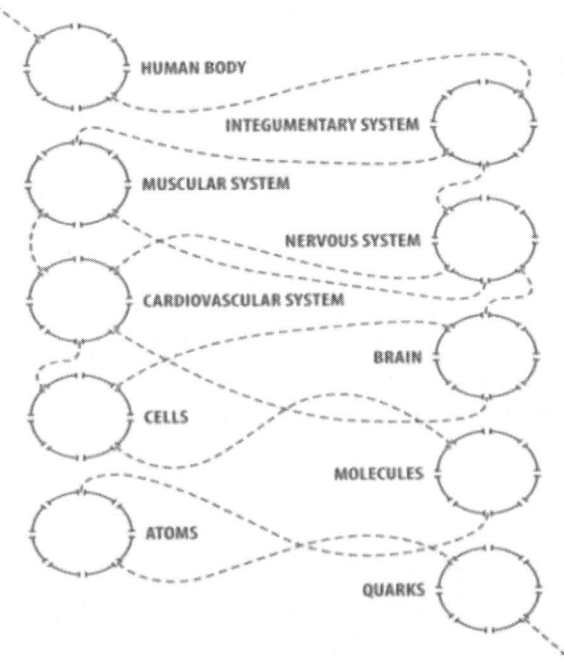

Figure 114. The human body.

The system of the human body consists of flows of packages between different subsystems, i.e., the integumentary system, S_i, the skeletal system, S_s, the muscular system, S_m, the nervous system, S_n, the endocrine system, S_e, the cardiovascular system, S_c, the lymphatic system, S_l, the respiratory system,

S_r, the digestive system, S_d, the urinary system, S_u and the reproductive system, S_{re}.

The flow of packages will over time change each of a, b, R and aRb. At t_1 the structure and its contents have one appearance and at t_2 the structure and its contents have another appearance.

When we apply the principle to the human body, the hierarchy of flows can be illustrated as below:

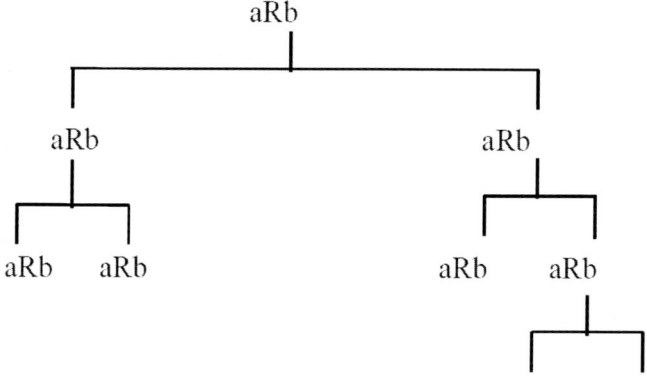

Figure 115. Hierarchy of flows within the human body.

Now we must identify all a, R and b, which leads us to this table:

$R_1 =$	$a_1 =$	$b_1 =$
$R_2 =$	$a_2 =$	$b_2 =$
$R_3 =$	$a_3 =$	$b_3 =$

And so on for billions of billions of a, b and R within the human body. **R** contains p_{1-n} and the function of R is as below:

$$R = \sum p_{1-n} = p_1 + p_2 + p_3 \ldots p_n$$

This content will over time change any structure a, b, c in the human body, from the lowest element in the cells to relations between subsystems. Within the body there are a complex R_{1-n}.

If S_H stands for the system of the human body, then

$S_H = (aRb)^{-\infty}$ consists of S_i, S_s, S_m, S_c, S_l, S_r, S_d, S_u, S_{re}, S_n and S_e, where each S_{1-11} has its own system of R_{1-10}.

$$S_H = (aRb)^{-\infty} = S_iR_1S_mR_2S_c\,R_3S_lR_4S_rR_5S_dR_6S_uR_7S_{re}R_8S_nR_9S_e\,R_{10}S_s$$

Based on the postulates and the Principle $X = aRb$, we can look into the system of the human body.

With the language of the principle of relation we can summarize the system, S, for the human body, H, as

$$S_H = (aRb)^{-\infty}$$

Since there are 100.000.000.000.000 cells, i.e., 100 trillion cells, where each cell is a living unit, between all cells and organs there are billions and billions of relations, R.

The human body is a complex system of relations between subsystems, down to the smallest elements in and between cells.

When any R is broken or damaged, there will be a disorder and disease.

Research has clarified how cells shuttle molecules, how vital chemicals are transported within and between cells, how the vesicles contain and release these chemicals and find the right destinations and release the chemical in the right place. Now we have to identify R_{1-10} *between* S_{1-11} and all R_{1-n} *within* all S_{1-11}.

Epilogue

Understanding reality is demanding, tricky and difficult.

By using established theories, we make it rather easy for ourselves. Even if we slightly expand our knowledge, for the benefit to humankind, we are imprisoned in these paradigms.

Galileo Galilei met the pope and the people of the Vatican during the seventeenth century and was advised to abandon the idea of heliocentrism. We have all heard the words *"Eppur si muove,"* i.e., *"And yet it moves,"* as we have been told that Galileo Galilei muttered.

Of course this cannot happen in our time. Or could it? Are we also imprisoned in existing paradigms?

I do not know.

Maybe.

But using an analogy of Galileo Galilei - *And yet flows dominate reality*, i.e., *Et tamen fluit re dominari* – an alternative answer might be given.

The method for examining and understanding the foundation of reality is simple:

- There are always established ways that describe reality. These cannot be used. They must be left.
- Then your own point of view must be formulated.
- The new theory cannot be judged by using established theories.

Thus, we can either use established theories and views of the world or we need to start from point zero.

If we use the equations of relativity, we know the answers.

If we use the equations of quantum, we know the answers.

If we use the theory of evolution, we know the answers.

If we use the theory of DNA, we know the answers.

And so on.

Taking the next step demands new premises and new angles of reality.

It is exciting, but lonely.

Meantime these quotes give us support and courage:

"It is the lone worker who makes the first advance in a subject; the details may be worked out by a team, but the prime idea is due to enterprise, thought, and perception of an individual."
Alexander Fleming (1881-1955)

"To avoid criticism say nothing, do nothing, be nothing."
Aristotle (384 BC – 322 BC)

"Do not fear to be eccentric in opinion, for every opinion now accepted was once eccentric."
Bertrand Russell (1872-1970)

"Every individual ... has to retain his way of thinking if he does not want to get lost in the maze of possibilities. However, nobody is sure of having the right road, me the least."
Albert Einstein, May 25, 1953

"What really make science grow are new ideas, including false ideas."
Karl Popper (1902-1994)

"The mere formulation of a problem is often far more essential than its solution, which may be merely a matter of mathematical or experimental skill. To raise new questions, new possibilities, to regard old problems from a new angle requires creative imagination and marks real advances in science."
Albert Einstein (1879-1955)

"Every great scientific truth goes through three stages. First, people say it conflicts with the Bible. Next they say it had been discovered before. Lastly they say they always believed it."
Louis Agassiz (1807-1873)

"New opinions are always suspected, and usually opposed, without any other reason but because they are not common."
John Locke (1632-1704)

"Three rules of Work: Out of clutter find simplicity; From discord find harmony; In the middle of difficulty lies opportunity."
Albert Einstein (1879-1955)

"No great mind has ever existed without a touch of madness."
Aristotle (384 BC – 322 BC)

"It has been said that man is a rational animal. All my life I have been searching for evidence which could support this."
Bertrand Russell (1872-1970)

"One of the symptoms of an approaching nervous breakdown is the belief that one's work is terribly important."
Bertrand Russell (1872-1970)

"My whole religion is this: do every duty, and expect no reward for it, either here or hereafter."
Bertrand Russell (1872-1970)

"I am my world."
Ludwig Wittgenstein (1889-1951)

"I act with complete certainty. But this certainty is my own."
Ludwig Wittgenstein (1889-1951)

Appendix I: Reality and the Paradigm of Relations

We are familiar with the existing views of the world of today, e.g., the theory of quantum, the theory of relativity, the table of elements, the standard model, different ideologies and religions.

The world is challenged by severe problems within societies as well as within science, e.g., nuclear weapons, population growth, refugee flows, climate change, starvation and diseases within societies; how to unite the theory of relativity and the theory of quantum physics, question the standard model, the table of elements and the theory of evolution within science.

Now it is time for a new view of the world - *the Paradigm of Relations* - that can handle and solve these problems. We must start all over again trying to find new answers.

In this chapter *The Paradigm of Relations*, based on *The Principle of Relations and its applications*, is demonstrated, since we need this foundation, which lies behind the new foundation of medicine. The paradigm overcomes established views and presents a new view of the world. For the sake of clarity some iteration is needed, then the paradigm will be coherent. The paradigm of relations is the springboard needed to climb to the next level of understanding reality, whether it is the human body or nature.

The Principle of Relations is based on these postulates:

1. "All" consists of the world today, the world of the past and the world of tomorrow.
    1.1. Everything that ever existed, exists or will exist is a part of "All."
    1.2. All is dynamic – All is "alive."
    1.3. All = **X**.
2. One world exists today.
    2.1. The world is a part of "All."
    2.2. Anything that does not exist today is not part of this world.
    2.3. The world is dynamic – the world is "alive."

3. Any world is differentiated into component parts, each one of which stands in relation to another.
   3.1. It all hangs together.
   3.2. Nothing exists in isolation.
   3.3. It all hangs together through a relation - **R**.
      3.3.1. Since it all hangs together, nothing is in isolation.
      3.3.2. The relation is superior to the parts**, a, b, c ...**
   3.4. If the relation is superior, there will be no cause and effect between the parts.
   3.5. The relation makes the parts' existence possible.
      3.5.1. Without relation the part will die and disappear.
   3.6. The concept of relation explains the concept of system.
   3.7. All systems are arranged in a logical hierarchy. If a superior system collapses, then all subordinate systems will collapse.
   3.8. All systems of relations, at a certain time, constitute the world.
      3.8.1. Everything happens only one time. - Nothing that happens will happen again. - The unique disappears and will never come again.
      3.8.2. Everything which is now will become something new.

4. Everything that exists is physically concrete.
   4.1. Meaningful concepts are concretely interrelated.
   4.2. Abstract concepts must be able to be derived from concrete concepts.
   4.3. The sentence expresses the thought in a way which is perceptible for the senses.
   4.4. There are no meaningful concepts without concrete meanings.
   4.5. The contents of thoughts are concrete.
   4.6. That which is concrete either exists or does not at a certain point of time.
   4.7. The combination of article 3 and articles 4.1 – 4.6 means that the world is alive.

5. Thoughts about concrete facts are meaningful propositions at a certain point of time.

These five postulates describe reality and mean that the concepts reality, the physical and the concrete are synonyms.

Based on the postulates we can now formulate the formula $X = aRb$.

Appendix I

The Principle of Relations, P_R, claims to represent all aspects of reality, based on I-III:

I. *Requirement for a complete theory:*
Every concept has to represent the reality directly and concretely.

II. *Postulate:*
Nothing exists in isolation, i.e., everything exists in relations.

III. *Basic concepts:*
1. Mass, i.e., m.
2. Wave, i.e., $\Psi(x, t)$.
3. Relation, i.e., p_{1-n} = flow of packages.

The concept of relation relates to reality by showing that there are relations between all parts in the physical reality, where:

1. **a, b, c** ... are any system, subsystem, unit or part in any field of the Universe, e.g., suns, planets, moons, galaxies, atoms, molecules, cells, organs and species.
2. The relation, **R**, is a flow (wave) of packages, p_{1-n}, e.g., quarks, protons, neutrons, electrons, photons, proteins, fats, polysaccharides, between a, b, c ... in any field of reality.

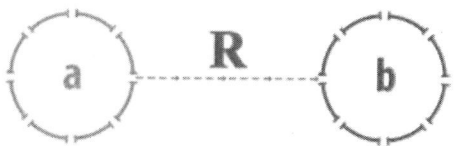

Figure 116. The basic model of relations.

Based on the postulate - nothing exists in isolation, i.e., everything exists in relations - in combination with 1 and 2 above, the principle of relations is **X = aRb**, where X stands for gravitation, forces, interaction and energy.

The same organizational principle rules at all levels, i.e., aRb organizes all masses and all matter at all levels of the reality.

For each level and for each system there are different masses/matter, and for each level and for each system adequate masses/matter occur. So, the atom uses quarks and leptons when an atom occurs and the solar system uses the Sun, planets and moons when it occurs.

In the Universe continuous flows of packages go in "tubes" between all systems, resulting in gravitation, force and energy. These flows contain all mass in the Universe, including dark matter and dark energy. The key concepts are flows of packages, gates, transformers and systems.

When any flow of packages arrives at any system there are gates transforming the content to fit in to the system, and then the content will change appearance.

A Transformer is *the mechanism which directs and leads packages*, e.g., protons, electrons and nutrient molecules, within the cells in the human body.

Throughout reality the same principle applies to the mechanisms of a Transformer's functions, e.g., the Earth, the Sun, the Moon, the human body, galaxies, organs and cells.

Please accept this simple illustration, where A, B, C and D are planets, suns and galaxies as well as atoms, molecules and conglomerates of molecules and cells:

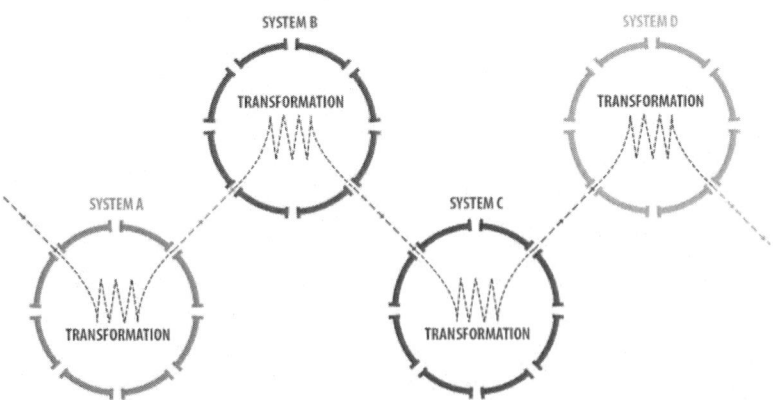

Figure 117. The model of systems transformations.

For each system there are gates, i.e., the transformation mechanism by the Transformer, where the content of the packages is transformed for the next level of physical reality.

Appendix I

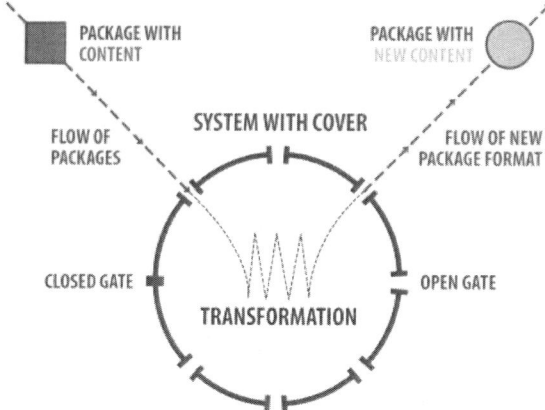

Figure 118. Emission and absorption of masses.

The basic structure of the Transformer can be presented by the following image:

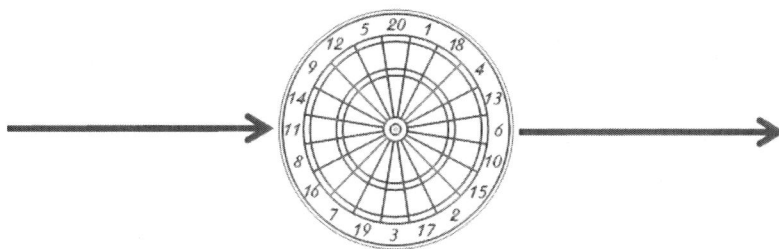

Figure 119. The Transformer.

A Transformer is *the mechanism which directs and leads packages*, e.g., protons, electrons and nutrient molecules, within the cells in the human body.

Throughout reality the same principle mechanism of a transformer is at work, e.g., the Earth, the Sun, the Moon, the Human Body, galaxies, organs and cells in the Human Body.

Once we have identified the Transformer and the flows in all parts of reality, we know how the Universe, the Earth, the Nature, the Society and the Human Body behave.

Since reality is based on *simplicity*, there cannot be any other answer than *one basic principle for the entire reality*.

The Principle of Relations and Its Applications

Now we must find out what happens when we imply the principle to different parts of reality, i.e.:

I. Logic
II. Physics
III. Chemistry
IV. Medicine
V. Biology
VI. Society

I. The Principle of Relations Applied to Logic

Now, let us find out the meaning of numbers based on the principle of relations. First number 1 and then number 0.

The Number 1
Based on articles 3.8.1 and 3.8.2 of the postulates, *a* and *b* change, which means that the content of *a* and *b* are different from time t_1 to time t_2.

1. $a = a$ at t_1 and this is called $= a_1$;
2. so a_1 is valid at t_1;
3. Then a_2 is valid at $t_2 = a_2$; etc.
4. $a_1 \neq a_2$;
5. $b_1 \neq b_2$;
6. $\Delta a = a_1 - a_2$;
7. $\Delta a = R$;
8. $\Delta t = t_1 - t_2$
9. Within a certain time $t_1 - t_2$, the content changes by $a_1 - a_2$ = content of R.
10. If $a = a$ at t_1, then $a_1 = a_1$,
11. thus $1 = 1$ at t_1, then $1_1 = 1_1$
12. if $a_2 = a_2$, thus $1_2 = 1_2$
13. if $a_1 \neq a_2$, thus $1_1 \neq 1_2$
14. Consequently, *a* and *1* are not static entities.

15. Thus 1+1=2 and a + b = ab is false, except at t_1; however t_1 exists before t_2, which is always the fact, i.e., what is true at t_1 is not true at t_2.
16. Instead we have to realize that at t_1 1+1=2, but at t_2 1+1 $\neq$2
17. This perspective gives a new interpretation to the definition of the natural number n, which so far has been defined as the set whose members each have n elements, which is a fallacy by circularity and therefore an impossible definition.
18. Conclusion 1: We do not know if the nature of the Universe is based on numbers.
19. Conclusion 2: Science, natural sciences and mathematics, based on the number 1, are not valid.

The Number 0

Up until now the definition of the number 0, zero, represents nothing; it is the symbol for emptiness, i.e., it represents the absence of any quality and its quantity.

But, since R exists, there is no empty space, whether in the cosmos or between particles, i.e., R is present with its contents all over space all the time.

Then, the number 0 does not exist and it is not valid.

The same conclusion can be found in this aphorism in Tractatus:

"4.128 The logical forms are anumerical. Therefore there are in logic no pre-eminent numbers, and therefore there is no philosophical monism or dualism, etc."

When Frege came to his conclusion, he first dealt with the concept's *unit, thing* and *object*; and if they are identical. "Why do we ascribe identity to objects that are to be numbered? And is it only ascribed to them, or are they really identical? In any case, no two objects are *ever* completely identical."

This is the question of unity and diversity, i.e., are numbers based on unity or diversity?

The answer, based on the definition of number 1 above, is that the symbol of any number, e.g., 3 will *not* look like this 1+1+1. The symbol 3 has to be shown like this $1'+1''+1'''$.

However, if the existence of arithmetic should persist, this is impossible, according to Frege.

How, then, can we deal with science based on the definition made in this paper?

We must invent *a new logic*, since the foundations of arithmetic are weak, i.e., *the logic of relations:*

1. $S_1 = (a_1R_1b_1)R_2(a_2R_3b_2) \ldots$
2. S is a complex of relations between all parts and elements in the system, i.e., the a, b, and c are complicated systems, that send and/or receive flows of packages, i.e., p_{1-n}
3. $R = \sum p_{1-n} = p_1 + p_2 + p_3 \ldots p_n$
4. The big challenge is now to identify all the p in all relations.
5. $(a_1R_1b_1)R_3 (a_2R_2b_2) \ldots$
6. $S = (aR_1b)R_2(aR_3b) \ldots$
7. $S = \sum (a_1R_1b_1)R_3(a_2R_2b_2)\ldots^{n-1}$
8. R_1 is the relations within the Earth; R_2 is the relations between R_1 and $R_{3-n} \ldots$
9. $(a_{1-n}R_{1-n} b_{1-n})R^{\infty-1}(c_{1-n}R_{1-n}d_{1-n}) \ldots$

II. The Principle of Relations Applied to Physics

Based on the postulate - Nothing Exists in Isolation, i.e., everything exists in relations – in combination with 1 and 2 above, the principle is:

X = aRb

Between all systems and between all parts of any system, S, there is a continuous flow of packages p_{1-n}, i.e., $R = p_{1-n}$. The formula will be this

S = ap_{1-n}b

Manifestations of the flow of packages are gravitation, energy, interaction, dark energy, dark matter and force.

Based on X = aRb and S = ap_{1-n}b any system is and can be described as complex flows. We might call them wave functions, since a wave function is a flow of masses.

We can transform the most important equations of force, relativity and quantum physics into the equation below, which unites force, relativity, quantum and energy with dark matter and dark energy, i.e.,

X = a ($\Psi(x, t) = p_{1-n}$) b

Where X stands for force, gravitation and energy, *a* and *b* are systems and p_{1-n} are a flow of packages.

Appendix I

The absorption of any flow of packages is guided by a *Transformer*, which is *the mechanism that directs and leads packages,* e.g., protons, electrons, photons and nutrient molecules, as shown in the example of Black Holes, i.e., Black Holes are Transformers creating new galaxies, suns and planets.

III. The Principle of Relations Applied to Chemistry

In the Table of Relations below, which replaces the Table of Elements and the Standard Model, there are many interesting relations for further research. For example, we can add atoms with other properties and reach an enormous number of atoms. The relations 1-27 are very interesting, but of course also the relations 73 and 46. Please feel free to choose the one you find most interesting. The table should be read so that each number represents one specific relation: e.g., no. 28 describes the relation between a proton and a molecule. Where can we find no. 28 in the physical reality? *Then the Table of Elements shows itself to be rigid and cannot represent reality.* Now, please feel free to use your imagination.

Entities, relations and system of relations									
Entities	Proton	Electron	Atom	Molecule	Cell	Planet Earth	Solar system	Galaxy	Intergalaxy
Proton	1	2	3	4	5	6	7	8	9
Electron	10	11	12	13	14	15	16	17	18
Atom	19	20	21	22	23	24	25	26	27
Molecule	28	29	30	31	32	33	34	35	36
Cell	37	38	39	40	41	42	43	44	45
Planet Earth	46	47	48	49	50	51	52	53	54
Solar system	55	56	57	58	59	60	61	62	63
Galaxy	64	65	66	67	68	69	70	71	72
Intergalaxy	73	74	75	76	77	78	79	80	81

Figure 120. The Table of Relations.

IV. The Principle of Relations Applied to Medicine

R contains p_{1-n} and the function of R is as below:

$$R = \sum p_{1-n} = p_1 + p_2 + p_3 \ldots p_n$$

This content will over time change any structure a, b, c in the human body, from the lowest element in the cells to relations between subsystems. Within the body there are a complex R_{1-n}.

If S_H stands for the system of the human body, then

$$S_H = (aRb)^{-\infty} \text{ consists of } S_i, S_s, S_m, S_c, S_l, S_r, S_d, S_u, S_{re}, S_n \text{ and } S_e,$$ where each S_{1-11} has its own system of R_{1-10}.

$$S_H = (aRb)^{-\infty} = S_i R_1 S_m R_2 S_c \; R_3 S_l R_4 S_r R_5 S_d R_6 S_u R_7 S_{re} R_8 S_n R_9 S_e \; R_{10} S_s$$

Based on the postulates and the Principle $X = aRb$, we can look into the System of the Human Body.

With the language of the principle of relation we can summarize the system, S, for the human body, H, as

$$S_H = (aRb)^{-\infty}$$

Since there are 100.000.000.000.000 cells, i.e., 100 trillion cells, where each cell is a living unit, between all cells and organs there are billions and billions of relations, R.

As we all know the human body is a complex system of relations between subsystems, down to the smallest elements in and between cells.

When any R is broken or damaged, there will be disorders and diseases, e.g., cancer, AV-block III, Alzheimer's and cardiac infarction.

V. The Principle of Relations Applied to Biology

SP is species, R is the relation between SP and Nature, N. N has impact on SP by R. SP will change as a consequence of N: s impact. With the language of the Principle of Relations we can summarize the change, not the evolution, of SP.

$$SP_\infty = (aRb)^\infty$$

Where a is N, which by R, i.e., p_{1-n} = flow of packages, will change b, to another species SP_2 or changes in attributes such as the size and shape of a species, e.g., the finch's pecker.

N → SP

$SP_2 = a_1 R_{1-11} \to b_1$

Now we must study how R affects the genes and how new mutations occur, *not as random events*, but as a logical effect of R, i.e., Nature.

S_{DNA} - the system of DNA.

aRb, where a is N, R is the content, i.e., p_{1-n} = flow of packages, and b is S_{DNA}

The formula is then $N_{1-n} R S_{DNA}$

VI. The Principle of Relations Applied to Society

Based on the postulate - Nothing exists in isolation, i.e., everything exists in relations - then the Good is actions that secure and assure survival and life quality in dependent relations.

When we directly or indirectly perform actions that secure and assure survival and life quality, we are doing good.

A world government is needed, based on a new constitution and a new pragmatic ideology for global politics, i.e., PASISM, a Power Assuring Survival of humanity, dealing with the global situation.

A comparison between 2021 and 2121 gives us what we need to do.

The world of 2021: the figure of $ 1.7 trillion represents global military spending for one year; nuclear weapons; population growth; climate change, nationalism, refugee flows, waste, democracy and its difficulties, starvation, diseases, corruption, false news, racism, migration, micro-plastics, decrease in trust, war, demagoguery, water shortages, conflicts, violence, populism, 193 national states and power blocs dominate the global scene, etc.

The world of 2121: disarmament and demobilization, forces for daily safety, food and medicine supply, access to energy, water supply, global equality, education, global infrastructure, legal and regulatory framework for the economy and business, laws and legislation, no waste, housing for all, and healthcare for all.

The image below illustrates the entire paradigm:

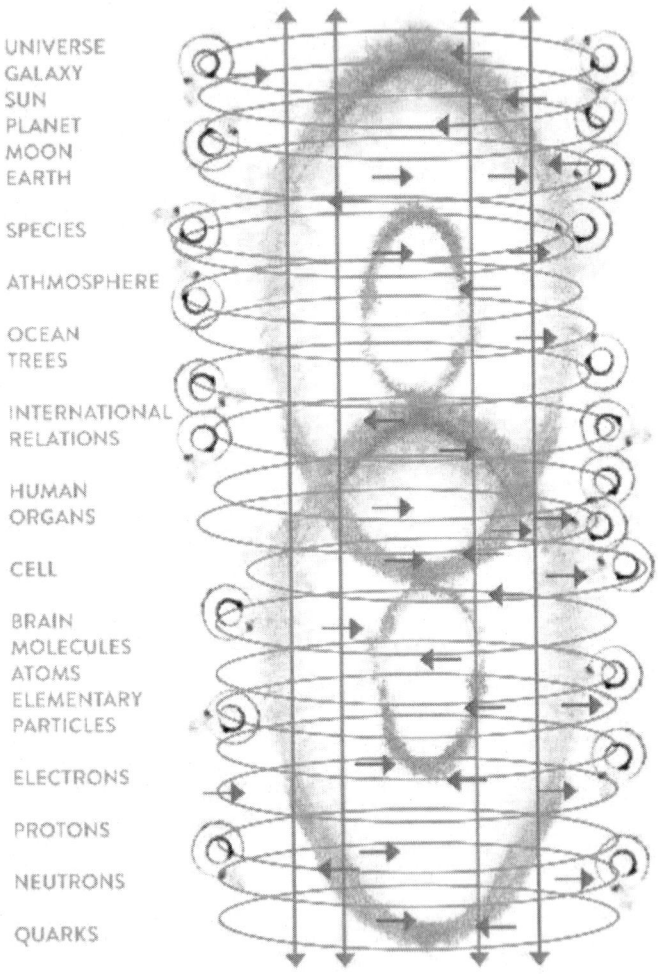

Figure 121. The entire paradigm.

Appendix II: Concepts Understanding Reality, Its Transformations and Its Different Shapes

The three most important equations of the past four centuries, understanding reality, are these:

1. Newton's theory of gravitation: $F = Gm_1 \times m_2/r^2$
2. Einstein's theory of energy: $E = mc^2$
3. Einstein's theory of gravitation, simplified: $G\mu\upsilon = 8\pi T\mu\upsilon$

These equations will now be replaced by the formula $X = aRb$.

By using five basic concepts, i.e., mass, flow, relation, transformer and shape, this new view of the world has been found understanding reality. These concepts are sufficiently and necessary understanding reality:

1. Mass
2. Flow
3. Relation
4. Transformer
5. Shape

Basically three dominant stipulated postulates are used:

1. Nothing exists in isolation; everything exists in relations.
2. Movement is a property of reality.
3. Every concept has to represent reality directly and concretely.

Based on postulate 1, the fundamental concepts and the fundamental equations will be the following:

The concept relation relates to reality by showing that there are relations between all parts in reality, where:

1. **a, b, c** ... are any system, subsystem, unit or part in any field of relation in Universe, e.g., suns, planets, moons, galaxies, atoms, molecules, cells, organs and species.
2. The relation, **R,** is a flow (wave) of packages, p_{1-n}, e.g., quarks, protons, neutrons, electrons, photons, proteins, fats, polysaccharides, between a, b, c ... in any field of reality.

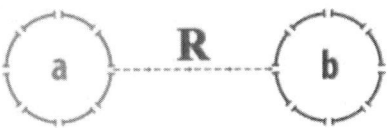

Figure 122. The basic model of relations.

Based on the postulate – *nothing exists in isolation, everything exists in relations* – in combination with 1 and 2 above, the principle is

$X = aRb$

The Principle of Relations claims that between all systems and between all parts of any system, S, there is a continuous flow of packages p_{1-n}, i.e., in aRb, $R = p_{1-n}$, and thus the formula is

$S = ap_{1-n}b$

S is a complex of relations between all parts and elements in the system, i.e., the a, b, and c are complicated systems, which send and/or receive flows of packages, i.e., p_{1-n}:

$R = \sum p_{1-n} = p_1 + p_2 + p_3 \ldots p_n$

The big challenge is now to identify all the *p* in all relations and to identify, certainly and concretely, the logic of

$S_1 = (a_1R_1b_1)\ R_2\ (a_2R_3b_2) \ldots$

Flows of packages are transformed by transformers, ending up in new shapes, e.g., new galaxies, new species and new surface of the Earth.

Appendix II

Any flow of packages consists of masses which stand in relation with systems. From system *a* the flow of masses moves to system *b*. This is valid for all masses in the Universe, e.g., galaxies, planets, suns, moons, atoms and elementary particles.

We need to find out how the emission and the absorption of these masses of the systems *a* and *b* operate and function. Then gates are crucial and important, and they can schematically be shown as in these two models:

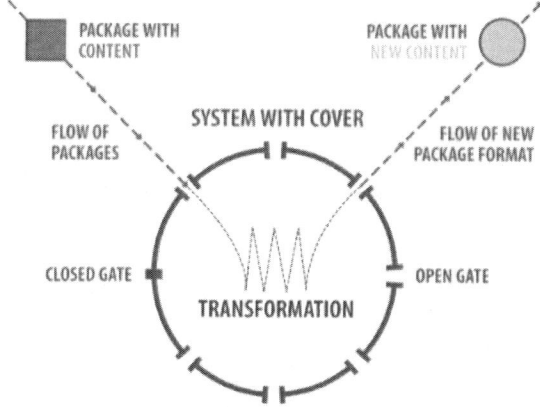

Figure 123. Model showing emission and absorption of masses.

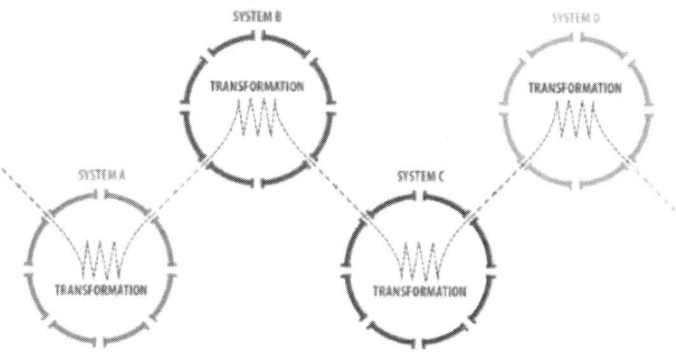

Figure 124. Model showing emission and absorption of masses *between* systems.

The Transformer of the Universe

Based on the basic model below, we can now imagine how flows are being transformed in the entire Universe.

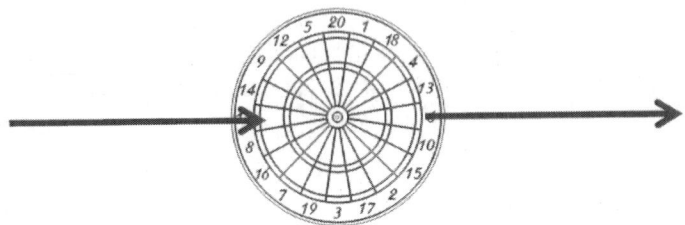

Figure 125. The Transformer in its basic form.

Then, let us apply these two pictures for the entire Universe, and with our imagination we can understand the complexity, as this model tells us:

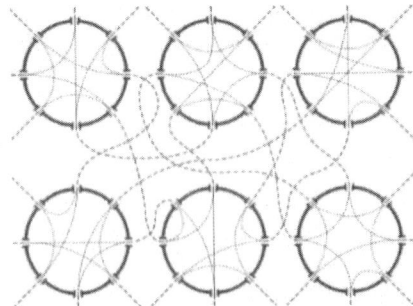

Figure 126. The model of reality.

The model shows how flows move between parts transporting packages, generating gravitation and energy, i.e., these flows are the foundation of reality.

Why matter occur in different shapes, such as the human body, a planet, a stone and the sun, has now to be focused. The Principle of Relations tells us how packages between systems function, but now we need to know why masses and matter occur in different shapes. We need to find out how and why different systems, such as humans, solar systems, planets, trees and stones are formed.

The questions to be asked now, is why a human has become a human, and why a tree has become a tree and why a stone has become a stone, i.e., why there are different shapes/systems in Nature.

Appendix II

Basically there is only one mechanism transforming masses to new shapes, i.e., *the Transformer*.

Let us now study the following transformers of reality:

1. DNA
2. Black Holes
3. Design of inorganic shapes

A transformer consists of the following:

Packages, i.e., p_{1-n}:

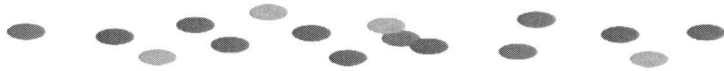

Pathway of flow:

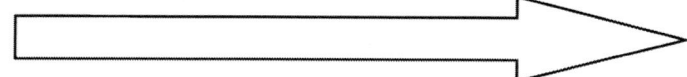

Infrastructure:

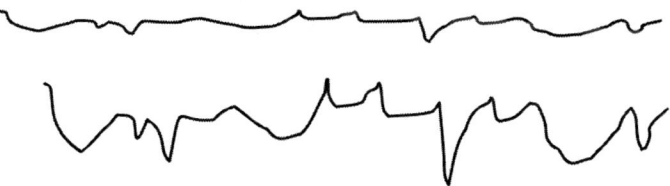

Figure 127. Three different parts of the Transformer.

There is interaction between the pathway, its infrastructure and the packages, i.e., they are weaved and interconnected together.

Packages enter the pathway in order, then by the infrastructure they are organized and transformed into a new shape; a new entity occurs, e.g., cells, organs, humans, galaxies, planets, trees, stones and water.

It can be summarized like this:

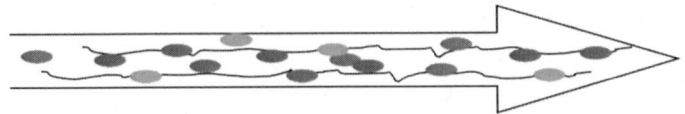

Figure 128. Complete transformer.

How DNA Transforms Masses

The Principle of Relations claims that DNA is an infrastructure, i.e., the mechanism which directs and leads packages of molecules, to be called *transformer,* i.e., DNA is a transformer transforming masses.

The Principle of Relations claims that the structure of the chemical components A, T, G and C organize how incoming masses are built. At a certain size, the cell has to divide, since it cannot handle to much incoming masses. Then, genetic information is the physical structure of the chemical components A, T, G and C. Even if sequences of A, T, G and C can be considered as a four-letter alphabet, it is concrete, solid and coactive chemical components, which allow flows to move in specific order, guided by the structure. When cells have to divide due to lack of space, new cells occur guided by the structure.

This will solve the problem of storing information, since there exists no information, it is the infrastructure of the chemical components, which automatically organize incoming components.

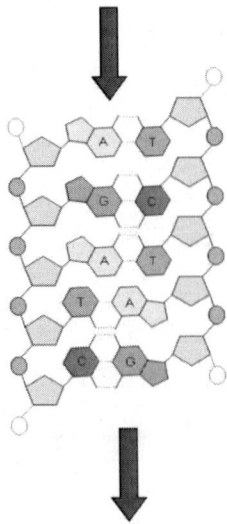

Figure 129. The infrastructure of DNA.

When flows of components arrive into the structure of DNA, they will follow the pathway within DNA, each taking its position when properties fit. Flows, consisting of chemical components, arrive and follow the infrastructure finding its place and position.

The model shown in Figure 129 is one example of the infrastructure of DNA.

How Black Holes Transform Masses

Black Holes might be "pumps" for flows of packages in the Universe, and a Black Hole might be a Transformer. They transform masses of packages into the next system in the Universe, e.g., Galaxies and Suns.

We need to identify and map all flows in the Universe and show how Black Holes function as the Transformers for these.

However, the principle of transformation via the Transformer is the same at all levels of the physical reality, e.g., between elementary particles as well as in the human body and in the entire Universe.

The equation of Black Holes is:

$r = 2Gm/c^2$

G is the gravitational constant, **c** is the speed of light, **m** is the mass of the black hole and **r** is the Schwarzschild radius.

The equation $E=mc^2$ contradicts Einstein's own criterion for a complete theory that *"every element of the physical reality must have a counterpart in the physical theory,"* since it raises the question as to which element the concept c^2 has in the physical reality. The argument could be made, that the equation then is not valid.

Since the equation $E=mc^2$ has impacts on the general theory of relativity, then this theory would not be built on solid ground. When c^2 is taken off, the Black Hole equation falls apart. What's left are the constants m and G, but they don't make sense any longer.

As for now, the equation for black holes is derived from Einstein's equation for general relativity:

1. Einstein's Field Equations, EFE, consist of ten equations constituting the general theory of relativity. However here I need to simplify the basic concepts in order to compare the concepts of the principle of relations.
2. The most used equation is this

$$R_{\mu\nu} - \tfrac{1}{2} R g_{\mu\nu} + \Lambda g_{\mu\nu} = \frac{8\pi G}{c^4} T_{\mu\nu}$$

Where the left side is Einstein's tensor and the right side is the energy-momentum tensor.
3. Working in geometrized units the equation is Gμʋ = 8πTμʋ, where G = c = 1.
4. To understand and elaborate the fundament of EFE, I will use the even more simplified equation Gμʋ = Tμʋ.
5. The curvature of space-time cannot be equal to matter/energy. It is not the amount or size of masses that creates the behaviour of the Universe, called the space-time curvature. An argument could be made that it is not as previously described but rather a consequence of aRb.
6. The equation must be GμʋTμʋ, which will now be seen as a description of the universe.
7. STCM means Space-Time-Curvature of Masses, i.e., STCM = GμʋTμʋ.

The simplified formula GμʋTμʋ can be transformed to X = aRb:

1. Gμʋ ≠ Tμʋ, i.e., mass and form are one in co-existing; it is GμʋTμʋ.
2. aRb results in gravitation by flows of packages, i.e., p_{1-n}, between bodies *a* and *b* in universe.
3. Form is the system where mass flows. Hence, the concept "system" replaces the concept "form" or any of its synonyms, e.g., architecture, design, space and shape.
4. What is left is RS, i.e., Relation and System, which is aRb.
5. From the equation Gμʋ = Tμʋ there are two valid concepts, i.e., mass, m, and form, f.
6. Then GμʋTμʋ is equal to mf, where m can stand for m_1, m_2, m_3 ... = p_{1-n} and where f can stand for form, which is the system, i.e., a_1, b_1, c_1 ...
7. Now we can translate GμʋTμʋ into aRb, i.e., $a_1 p_{1-n} b_1$.

Then, by using the equation X = aRb, we can transform the most important equations of force, relativity and quantum into the equation as below, which

Appendix II

unites force, relativity, quantum and energy with Black Holes, dark matter and dark energy:

$$X = a(\Psi(x,t) = p_{1-n})b$$

where **X** stands for force, gravitation and energy, **a** and **b** are systems and p_{1-n} are the flow of packages, i.e., $X = ap_{1-n}b$.

Simulations made by NASA's Ames Research Centre in California's Silicon Valley, using supercomputers, show how flows of gases between galaxies, i.e., the ebb and flow of gases, create new stars. The results of the simulations also show that space is not empty, which we know from aRb, and which we now know also with this proof. These results are supported by the Lyman alpha forest, looking like the so-called intergalactic medium.

Let us first take the position that the main content of gas (X) in the Universe is hydrogen (H), then in combination with the elements of iron (Fe), aluminium (Al), magnesium (Mg) and oxygen (O), we can illustrate the Transformer, i.e., Black Holes:

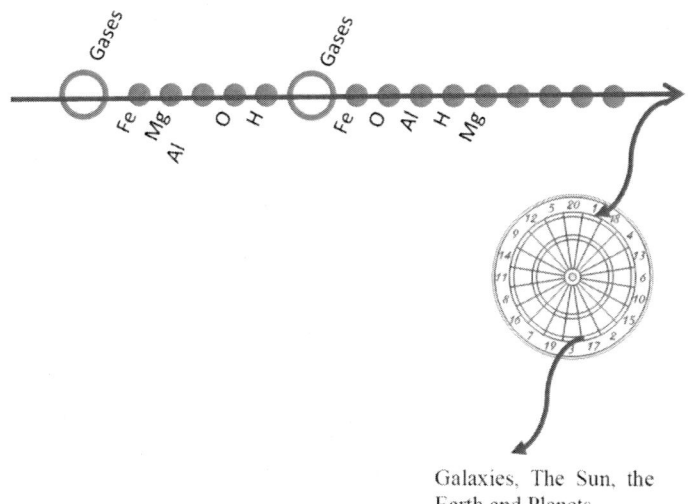

Galaxies, The Sun, the Earth and Planets

Figure 130. Black Holes as transformer.

Black Holes are Transformers between galaxies using packages of the so-called dark matter and dark energy. The conclusion is that Black Holes do not exist. They are only imaginary, based on wrong and not valid postulates and theories of physics.

How Transformers Transform Inorganic Entities - The Example of the Earth

The Earth changes, when R with its packages arrives via the "doors," i.e., the gates, of the cover. Crust, mantle, outer core and inner core are continuously changing the Earth by R.

Below is a picture, which illustrates the phenomenon applying the principle to the Earth:

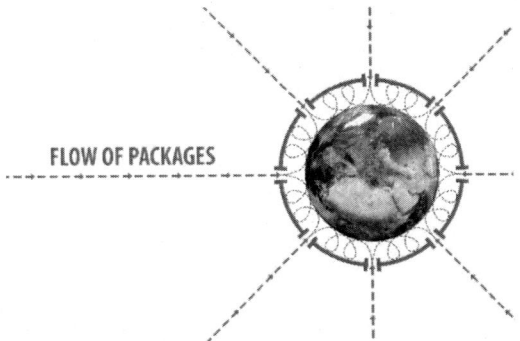

Figure 131. Flows of packages emit the Earth.

Then the following chain of events occurred; flow of packages affected Pangea, then the Earth of today arise and now flows of packages affect the Earth so that over the next 255 million years the Earth will change again.

Figure of the geological world 255 million years ago, Pangea:

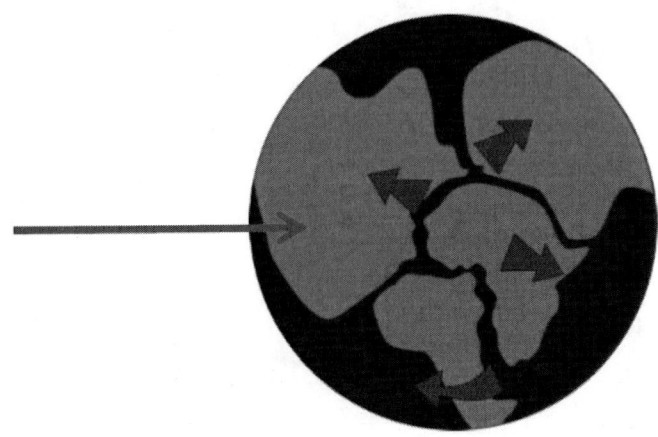

Figure 132. Pangea.

Figure of the geological world of today:

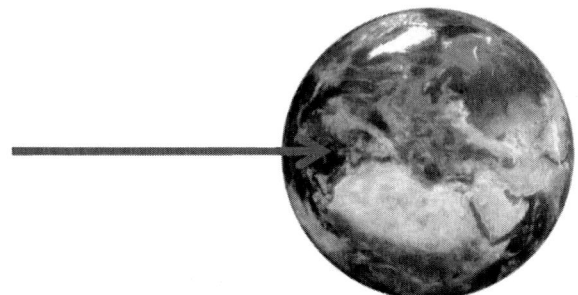

Figure 133. The Earth of today.

If b is the world of today and a is the world 255 million years ago, Pangea, then we have to find R, i.e., the packages that changed the world.

The continental plates move approximately six centimetres per year, as we know today. Then during the next 255 million years the plates will have changed position by 15.300 kilometres, since the plates move 1mm/week, i.e., 6 cm/year and approximately 0,5 cm/month.

The earths geological changes over time
The continetal plates change in kilometres

Yearly	Million years	255 million years
0,00006	60	15 300

We can now also make a probable picture, the figure below, of the geological world of tomorrow, Pangea Ultimo, 255 million years in the future:

Figure of the Earth in the future:

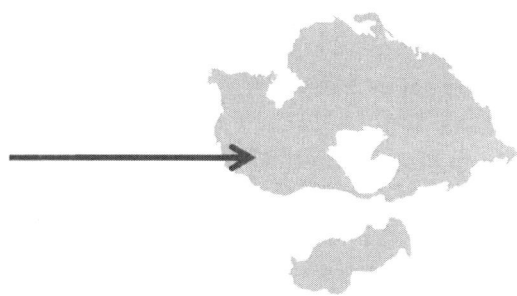

Figure 134. Pangea Ultimo.

References

A Brief Guide to Genomics (genome.gov).

Bernard, C. (1974) *Lectures on the phenomena common to animals and plants.* Trans Hoff HE, Guillelmin R, Springfield (IL): Charles C Thomas ISBN 978-0-398-02857-2.

Einstein, A., B. Podolsky and N. Rosen, *Physical Review,* Volume 47, May 15, 1935: *Can Quantum-Mechanical Description of Physical Reality Be Considered Complete?* Institute for Advanced Study, Princeton, New Jersey.

Gottlob Frege's paper *On Sense and Nominatum.*

How Does DNA Store Information? – CreationAndEvolution.org.

Raj Chovatiya and Ruslan Medzhitov, *"Stress, Inflammation, and Defence of Homeostasis,"* 2014, http://dx.doi.org/10.1016/j.molcel.2014.03.030, in Cell Press.

The Mechanical Mind: A Philosophical Introduction to Minds; Machines and Mental Representation.

The Nobel Prize in Physiology or Medicine 2013.

The Wisdom of the Body. New York: W.W. Norton and Company. 1932.

Thomas Nordström: *Are ATP Synthase and Black Holes Scientific Illusions?* (ijsr.net).

Thomas Nordström: *Concepts Understanding Reality, Its Transformations and Its Different Shapes* (ijsr.net), 2022.

Thomas Nordström: *DNA Transforms Masses* (ijsr.net).

Thomas Nordström: *How Mass Moves in the Human Body* (ijsr.net).

Thomas Nordström: *Reality and the Paradigm of Relations published 2021,* Nova Science Publishers, New York.

Thomas Nordström: *The Principle of Relations, 2018.* Cambridge Scholars Publishing.

Thomas Nordström: *The Scientific Illusion of Homeostasis* (ijsr.net).

Thomas Nordström: *The Theoretical Foundation of Medicine* (ijsr.net).

Thomas Nordström: *The Theoretical Foundation of Physical Reality,* authorHOUSE, 2020.

Thomas Nordström: *What is Inflammation?* (ijsr.net).

Thomas S. Kuhn: *The Structure of Scientific Revolutions.* 2012.

Besides these references, most of the material used is well known to all; they mostly belong to every man's general education. I use all material based on fair use and fair dealing, since it is in the best interests of science and that knowledge advances.

Index

A

ALS, xv, 13, 23, 24, 76
Alzheimer's disease (AD), 79, 107, 108, 115, 117, 118, 120, 121
ATP synthase, vii, x, xv, xvi, xvii, 16, 29, 36, 41, 46, 47, 50, 58, 63, 64, 66, 67, 68, 73, 77, 175
Attention-Deficit/Hyperactivity Disorder (ADHD), vii, 24, 123, 125, 126
AV node, 23, 124, 135

B

Brownian motion, 70, 72

C

cancer, vii, ix, x, xv, xviii, 3, 13, 23, 27, 34, 76, 78, 79, 80, 83, 84, 85, 86, 87, 89, 90, 92, 93, 94, 97, 98, 99, 101, 103, 104, 108, 127, 130, 135, 139, 142, 160
consciousness, 24, 126
cytoskeleton, 87, 88, 89, 110, 111, 112, 113, 114

D

deoxyribonucleic acid (DNA), vii, x, xi, xv, 13, 17, 18, 19, 20, 21, 22, 28, 32, 37, 40, 41, 42, 43, 44, 45, 60, 62, 80, 83, 84, 86, 92, 93, 104, 147, 161, 167, 168, 169, 175
diseases, vii, x, xv, xvii, xviii, 3, 13, 23, 24, 27, 30, 34, 35, 54, 75, 76, 77, 78, 79, 80, 84, 85, 87, 93, 99, 104, 108, 109, 112, 123, 126, 127, 129, 130, 139, 141, 142, 151, 160, 161
double helix, 17, 21

E

emission and absorption of masses, 7, 165
energy, 7, 9, 15, 16, 50, 57, 58, 59, 63, 64, 66, 71, 93, 104, 153, 154, 158, 161, 163, 166, 170, 171
extracellular material (endocytosis), 78, 87, 88, 110, 113, 114

F

flow(s), vii, x, xviii, 5, 6, 7, 8, 9, 11, 12, 13, 16, 17, 18, 21, 23, 24, 25, 27, 28, 29, 30, 31, 34, 35, 36, 37, 39, 42, 44, 46, 47, 48, 50, 53, 55, 58, 60, 63, 64, 67, 68, 69, 70, 71, 72, 75, 76, 78, 79, 80, 81, 83, 84, 85, 86, 87, 88, 89, 92, 93, 94, 97, 98, 99, 100, 101, 103, 104, 108, 110, 112, 113, 114, 121, 123, 125, 126, 129, 130, 133, 137, 142, 143, 144, 145, 147, 151, 153, 154, 155, 158, 159, 160, 161, 163, 164, 165, 166, 167, 168, 169, 170, 171, 172
flows of molecules, 16

Index

H

heart, vii, ix, 9, 17, 23, 39, 40, 68, 76, 78, 79, 123, 124, 125, 127, 129, 130, 136
hierarchy of flows, 12, 83, 145
homeostasis, vii, x, 27, 28, 32, 33, 34, 35, 36, 37, 39, 50, 59, 75, 77, 78, 133, 175
human body, vii, viii, x, xv, xvi, xvii, 2, 3, 5, 9, 11, 12, 13, 14, 15, 16, 17, 21, 22, 27, 28, 29, 30, 32, 34, 35, 36, 37, 39, 40, 41, 45, 47, 53, 57, 59, 63, 64, 68, 70, 72, 77, 84, 85, 86, 87, 91, 94, 95, 99, 105, 109, 117, 121, 137, 138, 139, 141, 142, 144, 145, 146, 151, 154, 155, 160, 166, 169, 175

I

induced fit model, 49
inflammation, vii, xv, xviii, 12, 13, 23, 35, 36, 37, 39, 75, 76, 77, 78, 79, 80, 81, 84, 99, 107, 108, 109, 118, 139, 175
integrin, x, xv, xvi, 13, 88, 89, 90, 91, 112, 114, 115, 116, 117, 118

K

kidney, vii, 9, 28, 40, 45, 78, 79, 86, 123, 129, 130, 131, 132, 133, 134, 136

L

lowest common denominator, vii, xviii, 13, 23, 86

M

metabolic pathway, 48, 51
metabolism, 14, 15, 16, 49, 51, 58, 64, 83, 99
metabolism of cell growth, 14
mitochondria, 28, 41, 45, 60, 68, 70, 92, 93, 104
mitochondrial dysfunction, 93, 104
MS, xv, 13, 23, 24, 76
mutation, 22, 43

N

neurodegenerative diseases, x, xv, xviii

P

paradigm, viii, 3, 8, 10, 27, 95, 105, 137, 142, 151, 162, 175
pathway, x, 9, 18, 23, 24, 31, 32, 52, 59, 60, 70, 85, 123, 130, 167, 169
plaque and tangle, 109
postulates, vii, xvii, xviii, 1, 2, 3, 5, 6, 12, 70, 73, 84, 141, 142, 146, 151, 152, 156, 160, 163, 171
principle, vii, xv, xvi, xvii, xviii, 5, 6, 8, 10, 11, 12, 13, 18, 22, 23, 27, 31, 32, 34, 35, 36, 37, 39, 40, 41, 42, 45, 59, 63, 64, 67, 68, 70, 71, 72, 75, 78, 83, 84, 85, 86, 87, 91, 97, 99, 107, 108, 109, 110, 117, 123, 125, 126, 129, 137, 139, 141, 143, 144, 145, 146, 151, 153, 154, 155, 156, 158, 159, 160, 161, 164, 166, 168, 169, 172, 175
Principle of Homeostasis, 37
Principle of Relations, vii, 5, 6, 10, 13, 18, 22, 23, 27, 35, 36, 37, 39, 40, 41, 42, 67, 71, 75, 78, 83, 86, 87, 97, 99, 107, 137, 139, 144, 151, 153, 156, 158, 159, 160, 161, 164, 166, 168, 175
process of transformation (transformation processes), 56, 57
psyche, 24, 125, 126

R

relation, xv, 1, 2, 5, 6, 12, 23, 35, 47, 60, 64, 66, 71, 77, 127, 129, 143, 146, 152, 153, 159, 160, 163, 164, 165, 170

S

SA node, 23, 124, 135
sodium-potassium pump, vii, x, xv, xvi, xvii, 16, 36, 41, 58, 63, 64, 65, 66, 67
suicide, 24, 76, 126, 127
system of flow, 36, 37, 59, 60, 77

T

Table of Relations, 159
testicular cancer, vii, ix, 76, 86, 97, 98, 99, 100, 101
Transformer, xi, 13, 14, 15, 16, 27, 29, 30, 31, 45, 46, 47, 48, 50, 53, 54, 55, 56, 57, 58, 59, 64, 68, 69, 72, 73, 75, 76, 91, 117, 154, 155, 159, 163, 166, 167, 169, 171
treatment, vii, 93, 94, 107, 120, 121, 129, 131

About the Author

Dr. Thomas Nordström holds a PhD in Sociology, having written his dissertation on decision-making and democracy in business companies. He has worked as Associated Professor in Entrepreneurship and Organizational Innovation Processes at the Blekinge Institute of Technology, Sweden, and as CEO at Research and Development Institutes, Sweden. He has written and had published several books and articles dealing with the theoretical foundation of science, see references.

Email: thomas@paradigmor.com